Understanding Mental Health Practice for Adult Nursing Students

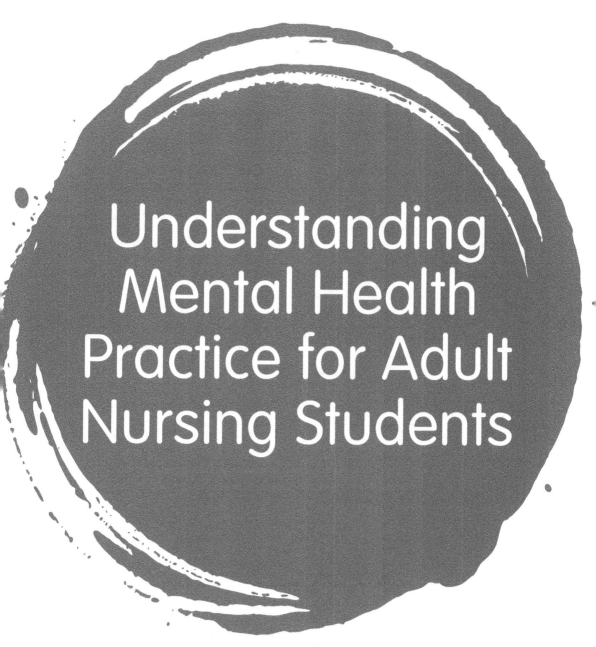

Understanding Mental Health Practice for Adult Nursing Students

Edited by

Steve Trenoweth

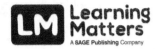

Learning Matters
A SAGE Publishing Company
1 Oliver's Yard
55 City Road
London EC1Y 1SP

SAGE Publications Inc.
2455 Teller Road
Thousand Oaks, California 91320

SAGE Publications India Pvt Ltd
B 1/I 1 Mohan Cooperative Industrial Area
Mathura Road
New Delhi 110 044

SAGE Publications Asia-Pacific Pte Ltd
3 Church Street
#10-04 Samsung Hub
Singapore 049483

Editor: Laura Walmsley
Development editor: Sarah Turpie
Senior project editor: Chris Marke
Project management: River Editorial
Marketing manager: Ruslana Khatagova
Cover design: Sheila Tong
Typeset by: C&M Digitals (P) Ltd, Chennai, India
Printed in the UK

Library of Congress Control Number: 2022930469

British Library Cataloguing in Publication Data

A catalogue record for this book is available from the British Library

ISBN 978-1-5297-1649-8
ISBN 978-1-5297-1648-1 (pbk)

At SAGE we take sustainability seriously. Most of our products are printed in the UK using responsibly sourced papers and boards. When we print overseas we ensure sustainable papers are used as measured by the PREPS grading system. We undertake an annual audit to monitor our sustainability.

Contents

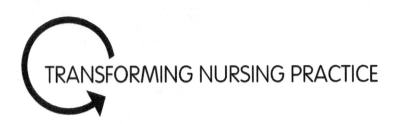

TRANSFORMING NURSING PRACTICE

Transforming Nursing Practice is a series tailor made for pre-registration student nurses. Each book addresses a core topic and is:

 Clearly written and easy to read

 Full of case studies and activities

 Mapped to the NMC Standards of proficiency for registered nurses

 Focused on applying theory to everyday nursing practice

An invaluable series of books that explicitly relates to the NMC standards. Each book covers a different topic that students need to explore in order to develop into a qualified nurse... I would recommend this series to all Pre-Registered nursing students whatever their field or year of study.

LINDA ROBSON,
Senior Lecturer at Edge Hill University

Many titles in the series are on our recommended reading list and for good reason - the content is up to date and easy to read. These are the books that actually get used beyond training and into your nursing career.

EMMA LYDON,
Adult Student Nursing

ABOUT THE SERIES EDITORS

DR MOOI STANDING is an Independent Academic Nursing Consultant (UK and international) responsible for the core knowledge, personal and professional learning skills titles. She has invaluable experience as an NMC Quality Assurance Reviewer of educational programmes, and as a Professional Regulator Panellist on the NMC Practice Committee. Mooi is also a Board member of Special Olympics Malaysia.

DR SANDRA WALKER is a Clinical Academic in Mental Health working between North Bristol Trust and Southern Health Trust. She is series editor for the mental health nursing titles. She is a Qualified Mental Health Nurse with a wide range of clinical experience spanning 30 years and spent several years working as a mental health lecturer at Southampton University.

BESTSELLING TEXTBOOKS

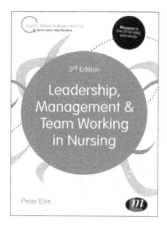

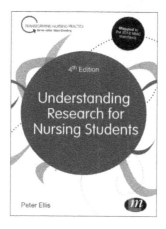

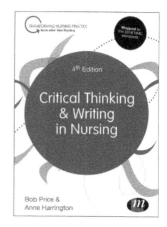

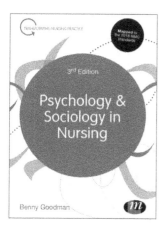

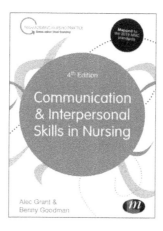

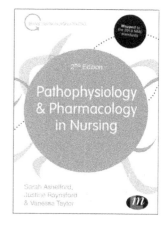

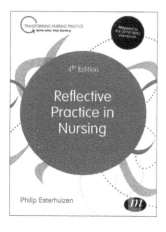

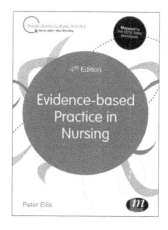

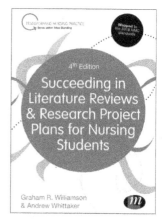

You can find a full list of textbooks in the *Transforming Nursing Practice* series at
uk.sagepub.com/TNP-series

About the editor

Dr Steve Trenoweth is a Principal Academic at Bournemouth University and was previously an Associate Professor at the University of West London. He has an interest in public mental health and is currently the Deputy Head of the Bournemouth University Integrated Wellbeing research centre (BUiWell). He has a particular interest in stress and wellbeing at work and has authored and edited many books and research articles.

About the authors

Dr Sue Baron is Programme Lead for MSc Adult Nursing and Senior Lecturer in the Department of Nursing Sciences at Bournemouth University. She has worked with international and national colleagues on research and education projects investigating simulation education and co-briefing (Canada, Australia, England and Scotland); student nurses' clinical leadership characteristics (England, seven European sites and Israel), empathy in health care (England and Australia); collaborative approaches to person-centred improvement (PhD, England); nutritional care practices (England) and health care experiences of people with learning disabilities (England). Additional areas of interest include innovation in education through co-creation, patient and public involvement (PPI); communication and interpersonal skills; palliative and end-of-life care and addressing inequalities in health care.

Dr Tula Brannelly is a Senior Lecturer in Nursing at Auckland University of Technology. She is a mental health nurse, researcher and educator with a longstanding interest in the implications of practice on people who use services, especially people who are most marginalised, whose voices are least heard, and who use the ethics of care to guide and review practice.

Chloe Casey is currently completing her PhD at Bournemouth University, researching the mental health and wellbeing of postgraduate research students. She is also a Lecturer in Nutrition and Behaviour at Bournemouth University, a Registered Associate Nutritionist with the Association of Nutrition, and a Graduate Member of the British Psychological Society. Chloe's research interests are wellbeing, mental health, coping and quality of life and the interplay with nutrition and dietary patterns.

Sonya Chelvanayagam MSc RN is a Lecturer in Mental Health Nursing at Bournemouth University. She is a dual-registered nurse in mental health and adult nursing and has worked in a variety of care services such as HIV, gastroenterology and pain management.

This has involved working with people who experience a combination of physical symptoms and mental health problems. She has published papers in gastrointestinal nursing, diabetes and eating disorders and interprofessional education. Sonya also works as a nurse in a day hospice.

Dr Zoe Cowie is a dual-trained nurse who then moved into education before retiring earlier this year. Her practice in mental health nursing was spent largely in the community where she worked for nearly 20 years in an ethnically diverse city. Since moving into education, she completed a PhD study on the stories of adults who were raised by a parent who has severe mental health difficulties.

Josie Tuck is a Lecturer in Mental Health Nursing at Bournemouth University. She trained as a registered Mental Health Nurse in 2006 and later went on to complete a master's degree in Advanced Clinical Practice. She continues to work clinically alongside her academic role in both community and inpatient mental health services.

Dr Sandra Walker is a Clinical Academic in Mental Health, working between Southern Health Trust and the University of Portsmouth, and is responsible for the mental health nursing titles. She is a qualified Mental Health Nurse with a wide range of clinical experience spanning more than 25 years.

Angela Warren has been coordinating PPI in the Faculty of Health and Social Sciences at Bournemouth University for the last 15 years. Using her background in education and drawing on personal lived experiences, she has been instrumental in developing innovative and engaging learning experience for students and promoting PPI in all stages of the research cycle. The inclusion of PPI in health and social care education and research is at the heart of all she does.

Foreword

We are whole beings. The days of blinkered thinking about body and mind somehow being separate and seen as disparate entities with little influence over each other are coming to a close. This truly holistic book shows us ample examples of research and practice that support a new perspective and help the reader to consider aspects of both physical and mental health as one and the same. As people, we all lie on a spectrum of emotions moving from periods of stability to periods of distress in response to various life events, trauma history, health, and so on. As you journey through this book, it becomes apparent that those in mental distress do not differ in any essential way from others, so thinking of people with mental health problems as different creates an issue that need not exist and feeds a stigma that helps no one. In the wake of a pandemic, the timing of this book is very pertinent and supports the societal upsurge in interest and understanding around our own mental wellbeing and how to look after it.

In this book, we have the opportunity to look at the concepts of physical and mental health, the practical application of law in the context of caring, care provision for those in mental distress and how to look after ourselves within this caring role. There are many practical exercises that will help you to develop a stronger understanding of the interplay between physical and mental health and think beyond the symptoms or behaviours you may encounter to the person experiencing them.

If you are a student nurse, a newly qualified nurse or even a nurse of some years' standing looking for tips to update your portfolio of skills, this book will stand you in good stead for practice. It can be read as a whole but can also be dipped into section by section as you come across situations in practice that warrant further exploration. Engaging with this book will help you to become a more effective practitioner of the art of nursing, enhancing your ability to care for people of diverse backgrounds and needs.

Dr Sandra Walker, Series Editor

Introduction

This book aims to give learners (and in particular pre-registration adult nursing student nurses undertaking BSc and MSc Nursing courses) an overview of the principles and practice of contemporary mental health nursing care focusing on the core knowledge, skills and values in supporting people in their recovery from mental health challenges. It demonstrates how theories, concepts and up-to-date evidence derived from nursing, social science and related fields can enhance the delivery of nursing care. Importantly, the book aims to illustrate how adult nurses can support the recovery of those experiencing mental distress and in so doing will provide a valuable resource to guide them through aspects of the new nursing curriculum which previously had not been covered on adult nursing programmes.

This comes at a time when mental health care has been under a spotlight. The recent National Confidential Enquiry into Patient Outcome and Death (NCEPOD, 2018), for example, highlighted a failure to integrate physical and mental health care which is leading service users with mental health conditions to receive poor physical health care. In particular, the report noted that general hospital staff lacked core skills and training in recognising and responding to mental ill health.

This book covers important and contemporaneous issues in mental health care, such as the concept of recovery from mental health challenges along with an appreciation of why the client's personal and internal frame of reference is so valuable within modern integrated nursing practice. In particular, emphasis will be placed on the personal process of recovery and discovery rather than on focusing purely on a biomedical model of disease and symptom reduction and medical/clinical outcomes, important though these are. For example, the reader will be guided to understand the importance of providing the right emotional and psychological climate within which mental health care takes place, as the collaboration and involvement of service users in their care are likely to be significant factors in their recovery. This is an issue which is of particular importance to service users, as involvement in their own care and having their own contribution to their recovery appear to facilitate recovery.

The personality, values and style characteristics of the nurse can be a significant factor in the facilitation of the recovery process. Thus, in delivering mental health care in diverse settings, nurses will need to engage in self-reflection, being mindful of their own resilience and emotional responses; capitalise on their ability to solve problems;

and be willing and able to engage with service users. This will also necessitate the ability to offer support to family and friends, as an individual's wider social network is likely to be a major factor in supporting recovery.

All pre-registration nursing programmes are approved by the Nursing and Midwifery Council (NMC) and are validated against their new educational *Standards Framework* (NMC, 2018a), which supports the integration of physical and mental health care. This means that in the new nursing curriculum greater emphasis is placed on developing more generic (or core) skills across all nursing fields, which are also applicable in various diverse and integrated settings. While there have been some elements of this in previous nursing curricula, the scope of the incorporation of mental health issues in the adult field will be challenging. Recent reports (for example, *The Five Year Forward View for Mental Health*: The Mental Health Taskforce, 2016) have also stressed the importance of health and social care integration, tackling stigma and discrimination, which will have the effect of lifting health and social care out of its 'traditional' clinical and professional silos to benefit patient/service user care and experience. Similarly, a recent policy focus on health promotion and ill health prevention, such as *All Our Health* (Public Health England, 2019), has found its way into the new nursing curricula. In short, what it is to be a 'nurse', and the context within which nursing is practised, is slowly changing.

Book structure

This book comprises eight chapters (summarised below), each of which highlights a number of key features of contemporary mental health care that are of particular relevance to adult nursing students.

Chapter 1: The importance of mental health care

This chapter, co-written with a representative service user, highlights the need for mental health care delivered by nurses regardless of branch or clinical context. The impact of mental distress on health outcomes (both objectively and subjectively defined) and the role of the nurse in improving overall holistic care will be highlighted.

Chapter 2: Integrating mental and physical health

There is currently a much greater awareness of the poor physical health care which people in mental distress experience. This applies both to those with psychiatric diagnoses and also those with physical health problems whose related psychiatric difficulties may have an important bearing on ultimate treatment outcomes and the trajectory of their illness. This chapter seeks to explore the importance of being able to adequately meet both the physical and mental health needs of people in mental distress. Changes to the role of the nurse in recent years will be discussed, as will the way in which the nursing profession can provide holistic care in diverse settings. An overview of essential nursing skills will also be highlighted in providing holistic care for the client in mental distress. In summary, this chapter will introduce why mental health matters in physical health care. It will establish the co-morbid links between mental health problems and physical illnesses.

Chapter 3: Understanding mental health problems

This chapter explores the various ideologies and paradigms which seek to explain the aetiology of mental distress (biological, social, psychological) and how these in turn affect care processes and treatment interventions. In addition to the medical model, social and recovery models of care will be discussed, along with various psychological approaches (such as behaviourism, psychoanalysis, and so forth). It will cover commonly encountered mental health challenges in physical health settings (such as those suffering from eating disorders, depression, anxiety, psychosis and dementia). This chapter will also consider the nature of mental distress as a complex phenomenon.

Chapter 4: Legal and ethical frameworks in mental health care

This chapter offers an overview of the Mental Health Law (such as the Mental Health Act (2007), Mental Capacity and Deprivation of Liberty Safeguards). Importantly, it challenges the reader to consider the nature of morality and how differences in lifestyle choices may be misconstrued as psychiatric pathology. It also gives an overview of ethical principles and dilemmas in mental health care and encourages the reader to use best available evidence, ethical principles and NMC standards and guidance to offer possible resolutions to complex case studies, such as consent. It will also highlight issues relating to inequalities in care, the impact of stigma and how the person with mental health challenges may be facilitated to have fair and equitable access to physical health care services.

Chapter 5: Supporting people with mental health concerns

This chapter will explore various strategies that could be employed by the nurse to help deliver person-centred mental health care. The focus will be on the skills of communicating and relating to people experiencing mental health issues or challenges. It will explore the *recovery approach* and how this can be used as a framework to underpin all nursing interventions, stressing the importance of partnership working and using a strengths-based approach. This ranges from general supportive care through to more structured 'psychosocial interventions' and in particular highlights a number of therapeutic interventions mentioned in the new nursing curricula, such as motivational interviewing techniques, cognitive behavioural therapy and de-escalation techniques. This chapter stresses the importance of engaging with the person who experiences mental distress and how effective communication, active listening and strategies for relating can support the development of therapeutic alliances. Essential skills of relationship management, communication and fundamental counselling strategies (again high-lighted in the new nursing curricula, such as active listening, skilled use of questioning, conversational and interpersonal skills) will be explored.

Chapter 6: Responding to a mental health crisis

In this chapter, readers will be guided through how to respond in a mental health crisis and what they can do to support a mental health service user at such a time, whilst main-taining their own safety and that of others. The focus in this chapter is to help readers to develop a more indepth understanding of mental distress, the ways in which it can mani-fest in people and how crises may arise. The chapter also supports readers in considering how to engage with those in mental distress and in building more knowledge of ways we can actively support people in crisis who access acute services.

Chapter 7: Overview of the therapeutic use of medicines in mental health

All students who graduate from the new NMC nursing curricula will be 'prescribing-ready' but may have had minimal exposure to the drugs that are routinely used in mental health care. Similarly, they may not have encountered some of the issues which arise for mental health service users, such as side effects. Good prescribing practice for mental health service users will be highlighted. This chapter will also explore the use of the Mental Health Act in enforcing medication, and the legal limits to this, whilst high-lighting the rights of people to refuse medication, and ethical challenges such as the covert administration of medication and coercion.

Chapter 8: Managing stress and promoting your own mental health

In this chapter, readers are invited to consider their own mental health and how this may be developed and enhanced. A discussion of stress vulnerability will be made, as will the notion of life events and ambient stress. Adaptive and maladaptive coping will be explored. The issue of resilience is one that features in the new nursing curricula, along with how nursing students can develop their own coping styles whilst adopting a mentally healthy lifestyle.

Requirements for the NMC Future Nurse Standards of Proficiency for Registered Nurses

The NMC has established standards of proficiency to be met by applicants to differ-ent parts of the register, and these are the standards it considers necessary for safe and effective practice. This book is structured to help you understand and meet the proficiencies required for entry to the NMC register. The relevant proficiencies are presented at the start of each chapter so that you can clearly see which ones the chapter addresses. The proficiencies have been designed to be generic, so apply to all fields of nursing and all care settings. This is because all nurses must be able to meet the needs of any person they encounter in their practice, regardless of their stage of life or health challenges, whether these are mental, physical, cognitive or behavioural.

This book includes the latest standards for 2018 onwards, taken from the *Future Nurse: Standards of Proficiency for Registered Nurses* (Nursing and Midwifery Council, 2018c).

Learning features

Learning from reading text is not always easy. Therefore, to provide variety and to assist with the development of independent learning skills and the application of theory to practice, this book contains activities, case studies, scenarios, further reading, useful websites and other materials to enable you to participate in your own learning. You will need to develop your own study skills and 'learn how to learn' to get the best from the material. The book cannot provide all the answers – but instead provides a framework for your learning.

The activities in the book will in particular help you to make sense of, and learn about, the material being presented. Some activities ask you to reflect on aspects of practice, or your experience of it, or the people or situations you encounter. Reflection is an essential skill in nursing, and it helps you to understand the world around you and often to identify how things might be improved. Other activities will help you develop key graduate skills such as your ability to think critically about a topic in order to challenge received wisdom, or your ability to research a topic and find appropriate information and evidence, and to be able to make decisions using that evidence in situations that are often difficult and time-pressured. Communication and working as part of a team are core to all nursing practice, and some activities will ask you to carry out teamwork activities or think about your communication skills to help develop these.

All the activities require you to take a break from reading the text, think through the issues presented and carry out some independent study, possibly using the internet. Where appropriate, there are sample answers presented at the end of each chapter, and these will help you to understand more fully your own reflections and independent study. Remember, academic study will always require independent work; attending lectures will never be enough to be successful on your programme, and these activities will help to deepen your knowledge and understanding of the issues under scrutiny and give you practice at working on your own.

You might want to think about completing these activities as part of your personal development plan (PDP) or portfolio. Once you have completed the activity, write it up in your PDP or portfolio in a section devoted to that particular skill, then look back over time to see how far you have developed. When you identify a weakness in a key skill, you can do more of the activities for that skill, which will help build your skill and confidence in that area.

We hope that you will find this book a helpful introduction to the key issues of mental health care and that you will feel empowered to help support those in your care who experience mental distress and who may be facing mental health challenges.

Chapter 1

The importance of mental health care

Steve Trenoweth and Angela Warren

NMC Future Nurse: Standards of Proficiency for Registered Nurses

This chapter will address the following platforms and proficiencies:

Platform 1: Being an accountable professional

At the point of registration, the registered nurse will be able to:

1.8 demonstrate the knowledge, skills and ability to think critically when applying evidence and drawing on experience to make evidence-informed decisions in all situations.

1.12 demonstrate the skills and abilities required to support people at all stages of life who are emotionally or physically vulnerable.

1.14 provide and promote non-discriminatory, person-centred and sensitive care at all times, reflecting on people's values and beliefs, diverse backgrounds, cultural characteristics, language requirements, needs and preferences, taking account of any need for adjustments.

Platform 2: Promoting health and preventing ill health

At the point of registration, the registered nurse will be able to:

2.4 identify and use all appropriate opportunities, making reasonable adjustments when required, to discuss the impact of smoking, substance and alcohol use, sexual behaviours, diet and exercise on mental, physical and behavioural health and wellbeing, in the context of people's individual circumstances.

2.5 promote and improve mental, physical, behavioural and other health related outcomes by understanding and explaining the principles, practice and evidence-base for health screening programmes.

(Continued)

(Continued)

Platform 3: Assessing needs and planning care

At the point of registration, the registered nurse will be able to:

3.13   demonstrate an understanding of co-morbidities and the demands of meeting people's complex nursing and social care needs when prioritising care plans.

Platform 4: Providing and evaluating care

At the point of registration, the registered nurse will be able to:

4.4   demonstrate the knowledge and skills required to support people with commonly encountered mental health, behavioural, cognitive and learning challenges, and act as a role model for others in providing high quality nursing interventions to meet people's needs.

Platform 7: Coordinating care

At the point of registration, the registered nurse will be able to:

7.5   understand and recognise the need to respond to the challenges of providing safe, effective and person-centred nursing care for people who have co-morbidities and complex care needs.

7.8   understand the principles and processes involved in supporting people and families with a range of care needs to maintain optimal independence and avoid unnecessary interventions and disruptions to their lives.

Chapter aims

After reading this chapter, you will be able to:

* understand perspectives of mental health, the changing context of mental health care and the implications for nursing education;
* highlight some of the assumptions that may be made about the needs and wishes of people who have a mental health issue;
* understand how important mental health is to our overall wellbeing and how the mind and body are not easily separated.

Introduction

In this book, we aim to help you as an adult nursing student to understand the impact of mental ill health on those for whom you routinely provide care. Assisting people to achieve a state of overall wellbeing is undoubtedly an important goal of nursing care.

However, adult nursing students often tell us that they feel ill equipped to provide support to people who are experiencing mental distress, and that they have a perceived lack of knowledge and skills.

Case study: Naomi

We will begin with Naomi, who has just started the BSc(Hons) in adult nursing after completing A levels in biology, English literature and maths. Her mother and sister are both adult nurses. For as long as she can remember, Naomi had always wanted to look after sick people and has had a particular interest in working with people who have respiratory issues. On starting her programme, she was very surprised to have a lecture from a mental health nursing academic who spoke about the importance of mental health and gave her group an overview of 'common mental disorders'. She was informed that under the new Nursing and Midwifery Council (NMC) Education Standards Framework, the scope of all future nurse practice will encompass assessment, care and intervention for people experiencing not only physical health conditions but also for those with mental health, cognitive and behavioural challenges. This gave Naomi pause for thought; she had not considered mental health issues as she had assumed that that was the responsibility of mental health nurses. She wondered if she would be able to do this and how she would be able to cope. She then remembered how many of her friends came to her to discuss their feelings or emotions and how comfortable she felt chatting about these issues. She also remembered how good she felt when she had helped someone to feel happier about themselves. Perhaps it might not be so difficult after all?

In our attempts to assist people to overcome adversity, which might be affecting the mental health of people we care for, we must understand the nature of mental distress. This is the starting point of the nursing care process – we need to understand the patient's experience and needs before we can intervene and provide care. You might think that the mental health issues are the responsibility of mental health nurses who specialise in the care and treatment of people who experience mental distress. However, the nursing profession as a whole is moving towards delivering more holistic care and there are expectations that adult nurses will be able to respond to the mental health needs of their patients, in the same way that mental health nurses will be able to respond to the physical health care needs of their service users.

Most people would agree that good mental health is important in our lives and that there should be health care services which support people's mental health and wellbeing. However, in the UK mental health has historically been the domain of specialist mental health services which have often been separated and disconnected from physical health care services (Attoe et al., 2018). We could be forgiven, therefore, for thinking that there exists a similar disconnect and separation of our minds from our bodies.

In this chapter, we will look at perspectives of mental health, the changing context of mental health care and the implications for nursing education and highlight some of the assumptions that may be made about the needs and wishes of people who have a mental health issue. We will illustrate how important mental health is to our overall wellbeing and show how the mind and body are not easily separated.

Service user voice

I felt there was a lack of attention given to my mental health needs whilst being treated in hospital for a physical health concern, particularly with regard to the administration and monitoring of my medication.

Changing health care services and nurse education

With the separation of health care services has come the separation of training to provide mental and physical health care. Nursing students in the UK have for many years had to choose from the outset a specific programme leading to a qualification in their chosen specialist field or pathway. The current NMC (2018a) *Standards Framework for Nursing and Midwifery Education*, however, goes some way to ensuring that all nursing students have access to all learning to take *into account the changes that are taking place in society and health care, and the implications these have for registered nurses of the future in terms of their role, knowledge and skill requirements* (NMC 2018a, page 3). For example, mental health nurses of the future will need to have enhanced knowledge of anatomy and physiology and skills assessing and caring for people with physical health problems. Similarly, adult nursing students will need to be able to assess and respond therapeutically to people who experience mental distress or who have diagnosed mental health conditions. However, while it is possible that nursing skills to support people experiencing mental distress may be developed, and the corresponding knowledge can be acquired across all fields, it may take longer for nurses to cultivate appropriate values, and to shed some of the assumptions about the needs of people with perceived mental health needs.

In many ways, the health care system within which you are practising is changing and this is connected to a different way of seeing the interplay between our minds and our bodies. Health care has traditionally seen that how we think and feel has no or little impact on the trajectory of physical illness and disease and that one can be 'treated' without the other (Attoe et al., 2018). But, just for a moment, imagine that you were diagnosed with a serious physical illness. Surely you would have some thoughts and feelings on the subject? And if those thoughts and feelings were profound this may have an impact in terms of our mental health. How we think and feel cannot easily be separated from what we do and how we behave. As Fransella and Dalton (2000, page 2) state; Each one of us is **acting** upon the world rather than **reacting**. That is, we actively try to make sense of our world. As we shall see in this chapter, the importance of our mental health for our physical health has perhaps been understated.

What is mental health?

Let's start by thinking about what the concept of *mental health* implies. We have noted in recent years that the terms *mental health* and *mental ill health* have been used interchangeably. For example, someone may say that a colleague is on sick leave because of their mental health. If we examine this more closely it seems not to make any sense – why would being *mentally healthy* lead to a person being on sick leave? Of course, what is meant is that the person is not mentally well, and it is very important to understand that the two terms (mental health and mental ill health) should not be used interchangeably in this way. Mental health is a positive state of mind; mental ill health is not. You may also note that we have not used the term mental illness – this is a contested term and seems to imply that a person is suffering from some form of disease. We must also consider that people may experience significant mental distress without being formally diagnosed with a mental 'illness'.

Activity 1.1   Reflection

What do you believe to be the essential features of mental health? Do you consider yourself to be mentally healthy?

An outline answer is given at the end of the chapter.

So, what do we mean by health, and what do we mean by mental health? As long ago as 1946 the World Health Organization (WHO) argued that illness was *not merely the absence of disease or infirmity*. More recently, in 2018, the WHO defined mental health as: *a state of well-being in which the individual realises his or her own abilities, can cope with the normal stresses of life, can work productively and fruitfully, and is able to make a contribution to his or her community*. It is important to realise that one does not *have* mental health – one has a *sense* of one's own mental health. The WHO definition recognises this when it states that mental health is when someone *realises* their abilities, and so forth. It is not, therefore, something which can be assigned by others but a personal and 'subjective' experience. We are mentally healthy when we believe it; when we sense it; when we see ourselves behaving in mentally healthy ways.

Service user voice

Mental health means to me, very simply, being able to get on with life as other people would.

Biopsychosocial perspectives

The idea that health and wellbeing encompass more than an absence of illness was proposed by Engel in 1977 in his biopsychosocial model of illness. Here, Engel argued that there is a need to identify how psychological and social experiences combine with biological factors to affect the course of illnesses. For example, how might the way that we think about ourselves and others think of us (such as in terms of discrimination, stigma and a lack of social inclusion) affect our health and wellbeing? Engel argued that there is a need to include a broader view of the *person,* as well as the illness, to develop a more comprehensive understanding of their health problems. These definitions of health and mental health take a broad view, seeing it not simply as biological dysfunction, but also a reflection of our ability to function, cope within and contribute to society. It is also very important for us to understand that not all people who experience mental distress have a diagnosed mental health condition and they may never seek or receive medical help for their personal challenges. Likewise, not everyone who has a long-term condition or health issue may experience mental distress. Today, we are increasingly beginning to understand the impact of childhood trauma or adverse childhood experiences on the development of mental health challenges, such as addiction, and the decisions that a person makes in their lives; see, for example, the works of Gabor Maté (in further reading, below).

In short, nursing care and our response to illness and the promotion of health are likely to encompass many different and varied aspects of the person's life and we must consider the *whole* person. We will look in more detail about what the whole person means in the next section.

Service user voice

I see my overall wellbeing as being able to function; not necessarily being able to hold down a full-time job but maybe being able to go out on my own; getting some independence back; both in terms of finances and activities of daily living. It's about being able to function to a personal standard I'm happy with.

The whole person

Activity 1.2   Reflection

Consider your recent clinical practice placement experiences. List the ways in which physical health care services seek to provide care to the 'whole' person. Can you spot any gaps in the services that they provide to their patients?

An outline answer is given at the end of the chapter.

Despite the broad WHO definitions of health, many have argued that we in the Western world have lost focus on the care and treatment of the *whole person* and there are calls for the delivery of care which integrates not only the mind and body but also physical and mental health services (Kunitz, 2002; Jonas and Rosenbaum, 2021). For many non-Western cultures, such as Islamic and Eastern religions, a holistic approach to life is an important concept (Rassool, 2000) and holism has been an essential component of the worldview of many ancient cultures, such as Australian Aborigines, Native Americans, Greeks and Chinese. However, for us in the Western world, there has been a separation of mind and body, with ill health seen to be an issue separate from the subjective experience of the sufferer. In the field of mental health, this thinking has led to the development of psychiatry as a medical discipline and the power and influence to control the response to perceived mental 'illnesses'. This involved the 'patient' passively accepting expert interventions and being subjected to coercive social controls.

Service user voice

I remember being compared to 'other bipolars' by a clinician in terms of symptoms, with little regard for who I was as a person.

Service user voice

My experience of psychiatry is one where my physical needs were disregarded. It's because they can't see further than your diagnosis ... They are powerful; they just ask, 'how are you?' and then medication.

However, there have been many challenges to this way of thinking. As mentioned above, Engel sought a 'biopsychosocial' model as a means of integrating the mind and body whilst recognising the social context of illness. Ludwig von Bertalanffy, who was to have an influence on Engel, recognised the complexity of biological and social systems, and more recently, James Lovelock in *Homage to Gaia* (2001) viewed the Earth as a complex, single and interconnected organism. There is also a political dimension to this. Medical sociologists, such as Ivan Illich (1975), have argued that an interpretation of ill health in purely medical terms attributes blame for an individual's illness or disease to factors located within the lifestyle choices they have made, rather than as a consequence of social and environmental factors brought about by industrialised societies.

The problem is that, in the provision of health care in England, there has often been a separation between mental and physical health care services and this has meant that strategies to improve physical health may not have sufficiently taken into consideration the interconnectedness between mental health and our overall health and wellbeing. Many have argued that there can be *no health without mental health* (Martin et al., 2007) and highlight that health services are often under-equipped to provide care for people with mental health issues and that the quality of care for people who have both mental and physical health conditions could be improved. They further point out that mental health awareness needs to be integrated into all aspects of the planning and delivery of primary and secondary general (physical) health care. A significant outcome of this way of thinking has been that people with long-term mental health problems, for example, often have had poor access to specialist health services where diagnostic overshadowing may lead to a misinterpretation of physical symptoms as psychiatric phenomena.

Service user voice

I was on a gastroenterology ward observing a young female (with a mental health condition) being treated differently to an elderly man; overhearing such comments from staff as 'Here she is again, it's all in her head'.

Mental health policy

In 2011, the then Conservative–Liberal Democrat Coalition Government published their strategy for mental health, which sought to improve outcomes not only for people who have existing mental health problems but also to *improve the mental health and wellbeing of the population and keep people well* (Her Majesty's Government/Department of Health (HMG/DH), 2011, page 5). In this way, this mental health strategy for England was as much about improving service delivery, staff development and the experience of care as it was about mental health promotion of individuals and whole communities:

> *If we are to build a healthier, more productive and fairer society in which we recognise difference, we have to build resilience, promote mental health and wellbeing, and challenge health inequalities. We need to prevent mental ill health, intervene early when it occurs, and improve the quality of life of people with mental health problems and their families* (HMG/DH, 2011, pages 6–7).

As implied by the title, *No Health without Mental Health* (HMG/DH, 2011) gave equal weight to mental and physical health, recognising that having a mental health problem increases the risk of long-term conditions (such as diabetes, respiratory and cardiovascular diseases) and early mortality. Likewise, people who have chronic physical ill health and painful debilitating conditions often have an increased risk of developing mental health problems (Margereson and Trenoweth, 2010). The guiding values of the strategy are explicitly recovery-focused and person-centred, emphasising control in helping people to identify personal outcomes, both physical and mental, that enable them to achieve a meaningful and satisfying life (HMG/DH, 2011).

More recently, *The Five Year Forward View for Mental Health* (The Mental Health Taskforce, 2016) recognises that physical and mental health are interconnected. The authors drew attention to the early mortality of people with chronic and ongoing mental health problems, with such people dying between 15 and 20 years sooner than the general population. Likewise, people with long-term physical health problems are more likely to develop mental health problems, which has implications for their recovery in terms of poorer outcomes. Medical science has, of course, been very successful in treating physical illness and disease. However, much of the success of medical care and treatment, of course, comes from advances in understanding the aetiology of diseases and from treating parts or systems of the body. While this helps us, perhaps, to treat a physical health condition, it does not help us to understand the lived, subjective or personal experiences of the individual who may be experiencing such diseases. This matters as there is much evidence that social, psychological, emotional and even psychiatric factors are implicated in the aetiology and trajectory of physical illnesses and associated symptomatology. There is also much evidence to suggest that good mental health promotes recovery from illness. This suggests a bi-directional model between mental and physical health and well-delivered holistic care, in which people who feel connected with and involved in their own treatment have better clinical and subjective outcomes (Hassed, 2004). The Mental Health Taskforce (2016, page 6) states:

> *There is good evidence that dedicated mental health provision as part of an integrated service can substantially reduce these poor outcomes. For example, in the case of Type 2 diabetes, £1.8 billion of additional costs can be attributed to poor mental health. Yet fewer than 15 per cent of people with diabetes have access to psychological support. Pilot schemes show providing such support improves health and cuts costs by 25 per cent.*

There is also a concern that the biomedical approach may create passivity amongst 'patients' who are seen, and may in turn see themselves, as 'ill' and in need of care, and as such:

> *Working from biomedical models encourages client behaviour related to boredom, lack of choice, disempowerment, fear, confusion, lack of self-esteem and confidence, to be perceived by nurses as symptoms of mental illness* (Rydon, 2005, page 86).

The recovery approach and personal perceptions of recovery

The growth of the mental health service user movement in the UK over the last 20 years has been dramatic, perhaps in response to the way in which mental health care services and psychiatry have often disconnected people experiencing mental health challenges from their holistic and personal experiences (Perkins and Morgan, 2017). Whereas there were only six independent user groups available for consultation during the drafting of the 1983 Mental Health Act, today service users are an integral part of mental health service planning and delivery at all levels. This increase in the influence of the mental health service user perspective has challenged many professional practices and, more importantly, the values that underpin these and has resulted in explicit consideration being given to the values necessary for appropriate nursing practice.

Today, the *recovery approach* is seen as a guiding force behind the mental health service user movement, and in creating a need for change in the nature of the relationship between service users and practitioners. In many ways, as it has been developed by service users themselves, the increasing influence of the *recovery approach* is an example of the success of service user involvement. Definitions of recovery here seek to recognise the impact of an individual's diagnosis and the subsequent journey of finding meaning in what has happened to them and discovering new sources of meaning and value.

The *recovery approach* stresses the holistic and biopsychosocial approaches whilst emphasising individual and personal pathways of recovery (Trenoweth et al., 2017). It does not seek to replace medicalised understanding of mental distress, such as those of psychiatry, but it places emphasis on the entire experience of the individual rather than a narrow frame of reference defined by a perceived 'illness'. The *recovery approach* also takes a different starting point to medical approaches in that initial consideration is given to how individuals may be assisted to achieve a life which is personally fulfilling to them, recognising their strengths, assets and abilities, rather than focusing on disabilities, deficits and symptoms.

Another, similar approach is the *Power Threat Meaning (PTM) Framework* (Johnstone and Boyle, 2018). Like the recovery approach, the *PTM Framework* seeks to understand the person's experience from their own perspective. It is a co-produced, negotiated understanding of mental distress, helping people to understand the sources of influence and personal meaning grounded within a social and interpersonal context. The framework helps people to share their personal narratives or stories of their experiences, as suggested by the questions below:

- Power: what are/have been the significant influences on you?
- Threat: how does this/has this affected you?
- Meaning: what sense can you make out of your experiences?
- Threat response: how have you been coping? What personal strengths have you drawn on? Who has been helpful to you?

The role of the professional nurse

The *recovery approach* represents, then, a set of values which has implications for guiding nursing practice and the way in which we work with and support people who experience mental health challenges.

Activity 1.3   Reflection

What do mental health service users want?

Consider the ways in which nurses might ensure their responsiveness to service users' needs in a modern and complex health care environment in order to bring about significant improvement in the health and wellbeing of those with mental health problems.

An outline answer is given at the end of the chapter.

Mental health service users have often pointed to the need to be treated in a 'human' way and with compassion (Khan et al., 2021). They identify the need to be listened to and to be understood (Shattell et al., 2006), and to receive a smile of acknowledgement; and to be given patient and empathic responses to their questions or requests. As such, nurses are needed to stand alongside sometimes frightened and vulnerable people to provide support and assistance to face, challenge and overcome the devastating effects of the issues which they are facing in their lives.

The role of professional nurses, regardless of setting, must be inextricably linked with meeting the individual needs of their patients, clients and service users. Rydon (2005) studied service users' views of the attitudes, skills and knowledge they felt mental health nurses needed. Service users expressed a wish for mental health nurses to convey positive attitudes in the sense of being professional, conveying hope, connecting with and working alongside, knowing and respecting the person and being interested in people's lives beyond their mental health issues.

Service user voice

Some nurses were polite, engaging with me. Sitting on the edge of the bed, just having a chat. Just basic human contact and empathy. This was important to me.

Rydon (2005) also identified a number of interpersonal and practical skills essential for the role (including exploring problems, using counselling skills, supporting the independence of the person whenever possible, and using organisational and teaching skills). Service users expect nurses to be demonstrably knowledgeable, in sharing their clinical knowledge and ensuring users are better informed about rights, and to possess personal resilience and emotional stability. Service users recognised the power imbalance between themselves and nurses and felt that, at times and under certain circumstances, this power could and should be used judiciously and in a positive way, for example, in protecting the person from themselves.

An important aspect of the *recovery approach* is that it stresses that to have needs is not abnormal (Slade, 2009; Trenoweth et al., 2017). The way forward in responding to the needs and wishes of service users is to recognise that service users want to be able to trust health care services, and have a decent place to live, money in their pocket, decent employment, friends, support, hope for a future, diversion from boredom; they want to be seen as a complete person rather than as a cluster of psychiatric symptoms and want comprehensive physical health care and assistance to alleviate psychological distress (Mortimer, 2006; Cutcliffe and Koehn, 2007).

Given the importance of the personal nature of an individual's experience of their own health, the measure of success of nursing care would be incomplete without an evaluation of its helpfulness from the service user perspective. Indeed, the best evidence of how helpful a nursing intervention might be is through the service user's response to, and satisfaction with, treatment and care offered. The service user is, after all, the expert on their own personal and unique experience.

Relationship formation

A central role for nursing practice is the development of the therapeutic and professional working relationship with those who seek our care and support (Cameron et al., 2005; Sheerin, 2019). Indeed, it is argued that the central work of nursing rests on the skilled use of the therapeutic self to promote recovery and to develop relationships with people who have diverse needs and, importantly, to be able to sustain such relationships over time (Peplau, 1952). Here, an emergent theme in the literature is the perceived need to *be* with people (Barker and Buchanan-Barker, 2011).

Of course, the formation of a trusting and therapeutic relationship and the creation of a positive clinical alliance are often seen to be essential precursors of effective nursing interventions. Indeed, service users who experience a therapeutic relationship appear to demonstrate a more significant improvement in their mental health and as such, the potential contribution to recovery is considerable (Hewitt and Coffey, 2005).

Furthermore, people who have significantly improved from mental health challenges have frequently reported that they were greatly helped by someone who believed in them; who gave them hope; and who treated them as individuals and not as symptoms of a disease (Cutcliffe and Koehn, 2007). Indeed, central to the process of relationship formation is the ability to develop respect for the others by getting to know, attempting to understand (Trenoweth, 2003), and empathise with, the service user (Cameron et al., 2005). Here, a fundamental requirement for the nursing profession is to be able to base its care on a sound understanding of, and respect for, diversity amongst people in their care (Üzar-Özçetin, Tee and Trenoweth, 2021).

Implications for adult nurses

So, today, mental health care involves concentrating on assisting people with improving the overall quality of their *life* and this may well involve helping people to manage the challenges they experience in their lives and to control their symptoms of a mental condition. In helping people to improve their quality of life, nursing care will need to be able to assist people, in a committed and compassionate way, to meet their mental and physical health and social care needs. Such interventions must be helpful in assisting service users to overcome their current difficulties but, crucially, must also be acceptable to them. Detailed information regarding treatment must be shared with service users and an explicit involvement in all aspects of care must be the norm. Individual care will need to be holistic (including an emphasis on responding to physical health care needs), bespoke and flexible, and provided to people from diverse backgrounds. So, as an adult nurse it is important for you to be aware of, and sensitive to, the concept of social justice, equal access to health care services and how they might tackle social exclusion and promote social inclusion. Above all, the adult nurse needs to support people experiencing mental distress in a human way and this is about the values that we hold as nurses and our personal qualities as human beings.

Chapter summary

In this chapter, we have looked at the importance of mental health care and the implications for adult nursing students. This includes being able to form and maintain helping relationships with people who may be experiencing mental distress and/or those who have a history of mental health issues. We have considered the changing nature of health care services, which now seek to embrace the whole person. Nurse education, too, has changed, so that the nurses of the future will be able to provide both physical and mental health care to people in a wide range of diverse settings, including forming therapeutic relationships and being responsive to the needs and wants of those experiencing mental distress and those who have a history of mental health challenges.

Activities: Brief outline answers

Activity 1.1 Reflection (page 11)

An important point to consider here is that people often confuse mental health with mental ill health, and it is not uncommon to hear people say that someone is suffering from mental health when more accurately it is mental ill health which is the challenge. The definitions of health presented here imply that mental health is a subjective assessment which encompasses our whole being – body, mind and spirit.

Activity 1.2 Reflection (page 12)

If you are working on a medical or surgical ward, there is every chance that you will have contact with different professionals who provide a wide range of physical health care (such as dietitians, physiotherapists, occupational therapists, and so on). Less common are those staff who are employed to work with patients who are experiencing mental distress. It would be a good idea to chat to staff to understand how they try to seek to provide care to the whole person.

Activity 1.3 Reflection (page 17)

Service users consistently tell us that they would like to be treated in a human way – by people who take their concerns seriously and understand their physical and mental health needs. The challenge, of course, in busy health care environments is to ensure that the whole person is looked after – this requires a combination of appropriate staffing levels, a culture which understands and respects the importance of caring for both the mind and the body and clinical leadership to make sure that the agenda of caring for the whole person is not lost.

Further reading

Frankl, V. (1946; 2004) *Man's Search for Meaning.* London: Rider.

A classic biography from Viktor Frankl, reflecting on his experience in a Nazi concentration camp, and how hope can survive under the most extreme circumstances. Life-affirming, inspirational and ultimately uplifting, despite its dark subject matter.

Maté, G. (2018) *In the Realm of the Hungry Ghosts.* London: Vermillion.

In this book, Maté seeks to explore the origins of addiction and the circumstances that promote human despair.

Wright, K. and McKeown, M. (2018) *Essentials of Mental Health Nursing.* London: SAGE.

An essential textbook for mental health nurses but also for adult nurses to develop their knowledge and skills.

Useful websites

There are many websites that seek to promote an understanding of mental health issues, including:

www.mind.org.uk/

www.sane.org.uk/

www.rethink.org/

www.mentalhealth.org.uk/

www.nhs.uk/oneyou/every-mind-matters/

Chapter 2

Integrating mental and physical health

Sonya Chelvanayagam and Zoe Cowie

(Continued)

Platform 4: Providing and evaluating care

At the point of registration, the registered nurse will be able to:

4.4   demonstrate the knowledge and skills required to support people with commonly encountered mental health, behavioural, cognitive, and learning challenges, and act as a role model for others in providing high quality nursing interventions to meet people's needs.

Platform 7: Coordinating care

At the point of registration, the registered nurse will be able to:

7.5   understand and recognise the need to respond to the challenges of providing safe, effective, and person-centred nursing care for people who have co-morbidities and complex care needs.

7.6   demonstrate an understanding of the complexities of providing mental, cognitive, behavioural, and physical care services across a wide range of integrated care settings.

Chapter aims

After reading this chapter, you will be able to:

- understand the relationship between physical health and mental health;
- recognise and understand the impact of mental ill health on physical health and poor physical health on mental health;
- realise the importance of holistic assessment and care and develop knowledge and skills to implement this in practice.

Introduction

In this chapter we delve into the connections between mind and body. To optimise the wellbeing and recovery potential of the individuals we encounter as nurses, being aware of a person's physical and mental condition is paramount.

The first section of this chapter will take you through the evolving understanding of how the physical and mental domains of being human are connected. This will enable you to appreciate how much more effective you will be as a nurse if you develop the skills needed to assess and care for the person holistically.

Activity 2.1   Reflection

Think for a moment and jot down what you think about whether and how the body and mind are connected. Are the body and mind connected? If so, how? Where do your thoughts on body–mind connection come from?

As this activity is based on your own reflection, no outline answer is given at the end of the chapter.

Rationale for the integration of physical and mental health

From the very beginning of our evolution people have known intuitively that body and mind are not separate entities. Some 2400 years ago, a Greek physician, Hippocrates (460–377 BCE) worked along with his students on the island of Kos. Hippocrates was so well thought of that he is referred to as the 'father of medicine'. The aim of the Greek physicians was to treat people holistically, i.e. mind, body and spirit, and so the treatment facilities included spas, massage parlours and temples where people would worship. Hippocrates believed that ill health was best treated with a good diet and exercise and only if that failed would medicine be given. Medicinal and mineral drugs were administered only on to the skin because Hippocrates believed that medicine taken orally might do more harm than good. This is where the oath in the *Corpus Hippocraticum*, 'first do no harm' – *primum non nocere* – originated, and it formed the basis of all future medical training (Ventegodt and Merrick, 2013).

Hippocrates was a highly revered man who believed in the healing power of love, therapeutic touch and honest processing of the emotions by talking. The belief was that 'not knowing who you are' underpinned all human problems so developing self-awareness and self-insight became the central tenets of healing body, mind and spirit, and the path to wellbeing. The self-exploration which was held to be so central became the role of the physician to facilitate in others. This meant encouraging patients to face and explore their emotional conflicts which were creating symptoms. This movement towards healing from the inside is known as *salutogenesis* (Lindström and Eriksson, 2005).

You will come across salutogenesis in your studies as it is a powerful construct which enables nurses to adopt a therapeutic and healing approach in every encounter. Without this knowledge there is a real danger that you might perform on a technocratic level only. This means seeing the disease or injury as the focus of your attention rather than the person who is ill or injured. Seeing individuals as more than their symptoms and being with them on their journey towards health is the aim of all nurses.

Concept summary: salutogenesis

Salutogenesis relates to the factors which support health and wellbeing (as opposed to pathogenesis, which relates to the origins of disease). The pioneer of this approach was Aaron Antonovsky, who proposed that it should underpin health promotion and public health research and practice. He believed that it is important to focus upon individuals' resources, their resilience and coping strategies, rather than their risks, disease and deficits. Salutogenesis can be seen as an approach which can be applied at the individual, group or societal level (Lindström and Eriksson, 2005).

Across the world, other health systems developed at the same time and in a similar way. You may have heard of Chinese medicine, which includes acupuncture and acupressure. In India ancient holistic medicine (Ayurveda) is also still strong today. Both ancient systems are founded upon a holistic appreciation of the individual. The Buddha (480–400 BCE), founder of Buddhism, explained that the mind and body work together, interdependently. Buddhist scholars are taught that the mind ebbs and flows like a fast-flowing stream in response to the bodily environment. The Buddhist practice of mindfulness is now increasingly drawn upon in current European mental health practice and is about attending to this constantly changing mind stream (Ventegodt and Merrick, 2013).

Very early Christian communities believed that human beings were spiritual beings: body and soul were one. Diseases were thought to be the result of personal or collective wrongdoing. It was also believed that for the soul to ascend to heaven, the human body had to be preserved intact. This mindset prevented the growth of medicine. It was not until the 17th century that French philosopher Descartes questioned these prevailing ideas and considered how the mind and body were interconnected. Descartes proposed that from a logical point of view, the mind and body cannot interact. His argument was that if the body is physical and the mind is non-physical, they clearly cannot relate to one another. A physical thing cannot interact with a non-physical thing. Like oil and water, the two will not combine. This led to what is known as 'Cartesian dualism'. Dualism is the view that the mind and body both exist as separate entities. To some extent this idea continues today.

The conceptual leap taken by Descartes, from early Christian belief to the separation of Cartesian thinking, enabled medicine to take some giant leaps. Essentially health became demythologised and for the first time anatomy and physiology could be studied. Separation of mind and body gave way to medical research based upon pathology and pharmacology. At the same time, however, separating mind and body denied the significance of the illness in an individual's experience of health (Mehta, 2011).

Dualism also laid the foundations for a movement where reality became based upon scientific, impersonal and unbiased observation and measurement. The person's subjective experience became separate. This means that objectivity was the only legitimate domain of research. This of course was a major shift in thinking and heralded the Age of Enlightenment (also known as the Age of Reason or simply the Enlightenment). It was an intellectual and philosophical movement which dominated Europe during the 17th and 18th centuries (Mehta, 2011).

The Enlightenment period generated a scientific revolution, particularly in disciplines like physics, chemistry and astronomy, which not only blossomed, but also came to define science. This afforded medical practitioners some scientific status, which eventually became viewed as the only legitimate path to knowledge.

Many doctors who were working with individuals displaying signs of mental distress became concerned that their status as doctors would diminish because social sciences did not lend themselves easily to scientific research, without running the risk of becoming dehumanised. This is when psychiatry was born. Doctors could then choose whether to work with people who were physically unwell or mentally unwell. The split between body and mind became deeper. The tendency of medicine to focus exclusively on the human body whilst disregarding the personal human experience has led to much dissatisfaction. Patients say they feel overlooked and disempowered because they are treated as though their body is a machine devoid of a sense of self (Mehta, 2011).

So why is this philosophy still in vogue across Europe? The answer is complex, but 300 years of investment in biological understanding which underpins the biological (or medical) model, as well as a good deal of money associated with big pharmaceutical companies, make redressing the balance unpopular. Medicine and pharmacology are extremely successful and powerful professions and so investment in research which might challenge some of the thinking is limited. People who do challenge this status quo are often seen as promoting unscientific nonsense (Ventegodt and Merrick, 2013).

In nursing, the idea that there is a separation of body and mind is associated with the view that there is something intrinsically dehumanising about the 'Cartesian' perspective because the implication of separating mind from body is that the patient comes to be regarded merely as a biological mechanism. One consequence of this line of thought during the past 20 years is that a lot of nursing theory has become anti-dualist, and anti-Cartesian. Cartesian-influenced nursing is now thought to be poor practice and academic nursing journals generally advocate for the reintegration of body and mind (Mehta, 2011).

Forty years ago, an American psychologist, Robert Ader, demonstrated how the immune system can be influenced by emotional states. His work heralded a new field of medicine called psychoneuroimmunology. Since then, we have witnessed an explosion of scientific findings. Research has led to the identification of the mechanisms which connect our physical health with our emotional health. There is now evidence to show how stressful emotional states alter white blood cell function. Stress weakens white blood cell response to viral-infected cells and to cancer cells. Interestingly, it is also now known that people who are stressed are less responsive to vaccinations and their wounds heal more slowly (Littrell, 2008). Ader has transformed the way we think about the relationship between life events, our environment and how our bodies respond biologically. Maté (2019) has highlighted how talk therapy can alter our immune response and improve the body's ability to fight disease. The chronic stress of poverty, for example, is shown to negatively impact the immune system. The evidence from psychoimmunology demonstrates clearly that although the mind and body were once considered separate domains, they are without doubt linked (Maté, 2019).

One major piece of work undertaken was the adverse childhood experiences (ACE) study by Felitti (2002), in which 17,000 people participated over the course of a decade. The findings showed that early-life experiences can leave an individual more at risk of many physical health problems later in life. These can include cancer, heart disease and immune conditions. The study provides a checklist of experiences which may occur in childhood: physical, sexual and emotional abuse, parental incarceration, parental alcohol and drug abuse, parental mental illness, divorce and domestic violence. There is a direct correlation between the presence of physical health conditions in adulthood and the number of ACEs scored. It was found that those individuals scoring 4 or more ACEs were 12 times more likely to have attempted suicide and experienced mental health problems than the general population. For more on this study, see the 2015 TED talk by Nadine Burke Harris, 'How childhood trauma affects health across a lifetime'.

The reintegration of the body and mind has been reflected in nurse education. In recent years adult nursing and mental health nursing have begun to reintegrate and there is now much more emphasis on the necessity for nurses to have a greater understanding of the interdependent nature of body and mind. Loving care and support are once again increasingly seen as therapeutic in themselves. Nurses are now increasingly educated to help human beings achieve health. This includes all the dimensions, from prevention of ill health to cure and the promotion of wellbeing. This means that nurses today must consider the human being, the environment and the health of the individual so that nursing interventions are truly holistic. How individuals think and feel about their health affects their experience, their treatment and their recovery (Todres et al., 2009).

Relationship between physical health and mental health

Activity 2.2   Reflection

Reflect on a time when you were physically unwell. Apart from your physical symptoms, how did you feel?

Did you become frustrated, frightened or low in mood? If so, why?

There is an outline answer at the end of this chapter.

Unexpected physical illness or poor health, whether short-term or long-term, affects wellbeing. Physical and mental health are interrelated in a number of different ways. Figure 2.1 demonstrates these biopsychosocial links.

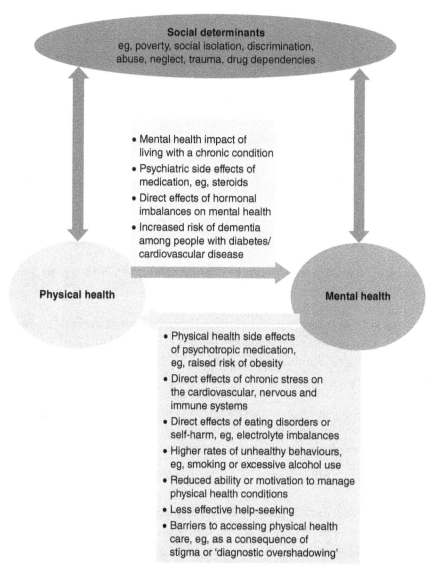

Figure 2.1 Mechanisms through which physical and mental health interact (Naylor et al., 2016; © The King's Fund 2016).

Understandable anxiety about the implications of physical ill health on both the person and family is common. The severity of illness – for example, whether this is a life-threatening illness, such as cancer – will detrimentally impact on a person's mental health. For some people this will be short-term as they adapt to their diagnosis but for others the distress is protracted, depending on how they adjust and their perception of illness. Coping strategies play a fundamental role as they help us to deal with everyday situations (Gross and Kinson, 2007).

When we become stressed or unwell our coping strategies can fall into two categories (Gross and Kinson, 2007) – maladaptive or adaptive:

- *Maladaptive coping:* difficulty in adjusting and responding in either an *emotional* or *avoidant* style:

  o *Emotional:* feeling miserable, depressed, and becoming frustrated with others, feelings of helplessness, believing the worst will happen and seeking sympathy from others;
  o *Avoidant:* hoping the situation will resolve, avoiding discussion and intervention as much as possible.

- *Adaptive coping:* adapting appropriately to the situation and learning from the experience in either a *detached* or *rational* style:

  o *Detached:* the person does not view the situation as a threat, does not take it personally but assesses and resolves it proportionately;
  o *Rational:* tackling the issue logically, using own experiences to problem solve and viewing the issue as a challenge that needs to be addressed.

When faced with coping with illness, Leventhal et al. (1997) stated people use these three stages:

1. *Interpretation:* understanding and making sense of illness; accessing illness cognitions. Changes in emotional states (anxiety) and coping strategies link to illness cognitions and emotional state;

2. *Coping:* dealing with illness:

   - *Approach coping:* active strategies such as taking rest, medical visits, talking about illness to alleviate anxiety;
   - *Avoidance coping:* denial of illness, wishful thinking;

3. *Appraisal:* reviewing effectiveness of coping strategies and deciding how to continue.

Additionally, involved in this process is the health locus of control (HLoC), which refers to a person's belief about their health. Rotter (1966) devised the concept of locus of control whilst he was researching people's expectancies of reinforcement or reward and whether they believed they had control over receiving rewards or punishments. Rotter (1966) discovered some people felt they had much control about whether they received a reward or punishment whereas others believed they had little or no control. He created the LoC scale and this has been further developed by Wallston et al. (1978) for use in health care (HLoC). These are the three categories:

1. Controllable by them: 'I'm responsible for my health' – internal LoC;

2. In the hands of fate: due to luck – external LoC;

3. Under the control of powerful others: 'Only the doctor can make me better/tell me what to do' – external LoC.

Individuals with internal LoC believe they are responsible for their health and therefore would be more likely to find out information about their health/ill health, attend health screening or engage in health activities (such as going to the gym) to maintain good health and prevent/reduce illness. In contrast, people with external LoC will believe that their situation is due to fate or bad luck and that there is little they can do to improve their health. They are very fatalistic in their approach to their health and will assume only an 'external' person, i.e. a health professional, can help them. Therefore, they seem to abdicate responsibility for their health on to the health professional.

This can help us understand why people respond differently to illness or a diagnosis, combined with their previous life experiences and current situation. De Vries and Timmins (2017) discuss the Moos and Schaefer model (1984) which includes these other factors.

People experiencing long-term physical illness, particularly cardiovascular disease (CVD), diabetes and chronic obstructive pulmonary disease (COPD), are two to three times more likely to develop mental health problems than the rest of the population (Dury, 2015). This can be due to the impact of their illness on their life, meaning they are unable to do certain activities maintain previous employment due to their physical symptoms restricting their activity, or their activity exacerbating their physical symptoms. Understandably this affects their quality of life (Vollenweider et al., 2011) but can also have financial implications which impact on them and their family (Mustata, 2019), and this in turn will affect their mood (Read et al., 2017).

Cardiovascular disease

In CVD, levels of depression, anxiety, panic disorder and stress are risk factors for a person developing this disease but are also experienced by a person living with the condition which negatively impacts on their physical health (Stoney et al., 2018). Severe depression increases the risk of mortality and stroke and has a greater impact on quality of life than the physical effects of CVD (Mustata, 2019). One-third of people who have a stroke experience depression (Cohen et al., 2015). They frequently also experience emotional lability; they become tearful and report a fluctuation in their mood with no obvious trigger.

When individuals are experiencing low mood or depression, they may lack motivation, are less physically active (Stoney et al., 2019) and their appetite is usually affected by either eating much less or more (comfort eating) than usual. They are more likely to consume foods such as ready-made meals as they lack the motivation to cook and prepare meals. Such foods are frequently high in fat and sugar. They may also experience a disrupted sleep pattern, which can have an impact on the development of CVD and mortality as their body is not receiving adequate rest and recuperation.

Case study: John

John is 55 years old. He is married to Jane and has two children who are 16 and 14 years old. He works for a building company and his job consists of heavy manual work. John has been experiencing some chest pain and breathlessness on exertion and palpitations. He is anxious and worried about his symptoms (which increases his episodes of palpitations) because his brother died at 58 due to a 'heart attack'. Despite Jane urging him to visit his general practitioner (GP), John prefers to manage his symptoms by drinking glasses of his favourite whiskey in the evening.

Activity 2.3   Critical thinking

- Why do you think John is reluctant to seek help for his symptoms?
- What coping strategy is John using?
- What are the implications of him not seeking help and drinking alcohol to manage his symptoms?

There is an outline answer at the end of this chapter

Anxiety can also precipitate CVD due to the physiological impact of ongoing arousal and the symptoms experienced, such as increased heart rate and respiration (Mustata, 2019). This is due to the release of adrenaline and noradrenaline from the adrenal medulla in the adrenal gland, which prepares the body for 'fight or flight' by diverting blood to the essential organs and increasing metabolic rate, heart rate and blood pressure and releasing glucose from the cells to provide energy to deal with the physical exertion required (Waugh and Grant, 2018). This is very effective for a short-term 'crisis', but not for a protracted period. Stress provides prolonged elevated levels of glucocorticoids. These are steroid hormones produced in the adrenal medulla which are essential for life and regulate metabolism as well as inhibiting the function of the immune system and responding to inflammation (Waugh and Grant, 2018). The main steroid hormone is cortisol. Levels that are elevated in the long term will cause prolonged immune suppression and the person will be more susceptible to infections (Cook et al., 2021) and also potentially cancer.

Chronic obstructive pulmonary disease

People living with COPD are three times more likely to experience mental health problems, particularly anxiety and panic disorder (Elassal et al., 2013; Breland et al., 2015). When you consider the symptoms of COPD and asthma it is not surprising that they may experience panic and anxiety. When caring for someone with an acute exacerbation of their respiratory symptoms, be aware of how frightening it can be for a person to have difficulty breathing and a fear of not being able to 'catch their breath'. Also remember that if a person has experienced a recent life event such as a bereavement this can make it more difficult for them to manage their condition.

Case study: Joan

Joan, 84 years old, has been admitted to the acute medical unit with a severe chest infection which has exacerbated her symptoms of COPD. She usually manages well at home with the support of her husband, but he died 3 months ago. Sarah, a second-year student nurse, is looking after Joan and notices that as well as her laboured breathing and increased respiratory rate, Joan appears very anxious. Sarah realises it will be an additional effort for Joan to talk but sits with her for a short time holding her hand (she is aware Joan responds positively to touch) and she notices that her respiratory rate decreases, her breathing is less laboured and Joan appears to relax.

Activity 2.4   Critical thinking

- Why may Joan be anxious?
- Why was Sarah's intervention effective?

There is an outline answer at the end of this chapter.

Diabetes

People living with diabetes – both type 1 and type 2 – are two to three times more likely to experience low mood, particularly in type 1 diabetes. If you consider how a person with type 1 diabetes has to manage their symptoms and that it will affect all aspects of their life, this will not be surprising. However, more recently it has also been discovered that as many as 20% of young women with type 1 diabetes also have symptoms of an eating disorder such as anorexia nervosa or bulimia nervosa (Chelvanayagam and James, 2018). Women with type 1 diabetes are twice as likely to develop an eating disorder than those without it and it can also be seen in men (Doyle et al., 2017). They tend to restrict or omit their insulin to lose weight and this may be accompanied by restricted eating and then consuming a large amount of food. They feel ashamed of their behaviour and will conceal their symptoms. Worryingly, they are more likely to experience frequent episodes of diabetic ketoacidosis, complications from their diabetes, and have increased risk of mortality. So, it is crucial that these symptoms are recognised as soon as possible to ensure they receive the correct treatment and support (Chelvanayagam and James, 2018).

Case study: Emma

Emma is 19 years old and has type 1 diabetes. The GP has requested to see Emma as she has discovered that Emma is only sporadically collecting her prescription and not attending appointments at the diabetic clinic. On further questioning Emma was experiencing polyuria, polydipsia and lethargy. The GP noted that she appeared severely underweight and malnourished. Emma admitted that she did not check her blood glucose frequently and has found that allowing it to run high and omitting her insulin have helped her to lose weight. The GP informed Emma that she is at high risk of diabetic ketoacidosis and complications from her diabetes and therefore requested urgent input from both the diabetes team and the mental health team.

Gastrointestinal disorders

People experiencing eating disorders may also present in gastrointestinal (GI) services with a wide range of symptoms such as early satiety, postprandial discomfort, abdominal fullness, abdominal discomfort and swollen salivary glands. They may also report diarrhoea, abdominal cramping and constipation. These symptoms form part of their eating disorder; however, the eating disorder also causes the symptoms (Chelvanayagam and Newell, 2015). They are frequently nursed on acute medical units although it may not be initially recognised that they have an eating disorder. They may not realise themselves that they have an eating disorder, or due to the stigma they may be reluctant to attend mental health services.

It is important to remember, as with all physical conditions, that as well as symptoms arising from the effects of their eating disorder, they may have an underlying GI disorder.

Case study: Faith

Faith, 19 years old, was being reviewed by Julie, inflammatory bowel disease nurse specialist, as she has recently experienced a flare-up of her Crohn's disease. The nurse was concerned as, despite Faith now being in remission and her symptoms controlled, she was very underweight, with a body mass index (BMI) of 17. When asked about her eating and weight Faith became very distressed and noticeably anxious, attempting to end the consultation. She suddenly burst into tears and stated that her friends had said, 'when you are unwell, you have a great body'. Faith had noticed when in the shopping centre that people looked at her when she was thin, but 'I become invisible when I gain weight'.

Activity 2.5   Critical thinking

- What would be your concerns in this situation?
- How can Julie help Faith?

There is an outline answer at the end of this chapter.

Interestingly, the GI tract contains a network of 500 million neurons (nerves), known as the enteric nervous system (ENS). Apart from the central nervous system, the ENS has the greatest quantity and complexity of nerves and it is sometimes known as the 'little brain' as it directly links with the central nervous system and links your thoughts and emotions to the GI system via the vagus nerve in a bi-directional manner, i.e. from your brain to your GI system, and vice versa. This is known as the brain–gut axis. The GI system responds to any psychological distress; consider the expression and sensation of 'I've got butterflies in my tummy' and 'gut feeling' (Dennett, 2021). It has been noted that the microbes which live within the intestines contribute to our mental health by way of the brain–gut axis (McEwen and Fenasse, 2019).

Conditions such as irritable bowel syndrome (IBS) are now considered to be a disorder of gut-brain interaction. People living with IBS are more likely to experience mental ill health such as depression and anxiety and report their first symptoms coincided with increased stress levels. They also have alterations in their gut microbiota (Dennett, 2021). Therefore, it is not surprising that some anti-depressant medications have been effective at managing symptoms of IBS and abdominal pain, as they manage the pain but can also help alleviate low mood.

Misuse of alcohol also has a direct impact on the GI system. It can cause chronic inflammation of the mucosa in the mouth and pharynx, which may cause pre-cancerous lesions. Nausea and vomiting may induce Mallory–Weiss tears in the oesophagus and stomach. Cirrhosis of the liver can cause oesophageal varices and subsequent bleeding and individuals can also experience gastritis and pancreatitis. However, the most common cause of liver failure is due to paracetamol overdose, hence the need to administer intravenous acetylcysteine when this is suspected, as it can be 100% effective in preventing liver damage if administered within 8 hours of the overdose.

Cancer

One in two people will be diagnosed with cancer in their lifetime and there are approximately 367,000 new cancer cases in the UK every year (Cancer Research UK, 2021). As with many chronic conditions, the highest rates are in the most deprived areas, with 16,800 cases linked with deprivation (Cancer Research UK, 2021).

However, the survival rate is increasing, and more people live with cancer. Despite this, when informed of a cancer diagnosis people will frequently express fear and feel helpless. Their response can be like a post-traumatic stress disorder and even when the cancer is in remission, they can still experience chronic stress and poorer quality of life. They may possess negative metacognitive beliefs such as 'if I cough my breast cancer will spread'. Such beliefs increase anxiety and cause low mood and may affect adherence to their treatment regimes. Research has shown that if individuals with cancer confront their stressor (cancer) and express how they feel, it helps with managing their cancer symptoms such as pain and inflammation, as well as improving adherence to treatment (Nejad et al., 2020).

However, a person diagnosed with schizophrenia or bipolar disorder is less likely to be offered a range of treatments and surgeries for cancer, due to concerns regarding mental capacity and drug interactions with their mental health medication (Fond et al., 2019). Their cancer diagnosis tends to occur much later (Donald and Stajduhar, 2019; Fond et al., 2019) so the cancer is usually stage 3 or 4 and therefore treatment will be less effective. They are less likely to be involved in preventive treatments such as cancer screening or offered interventions to stop smoking (Naylor et al., 2016). They may not engage in a care package due to lack of understanding, mental health symptoms or denial (Donald and Stajduhar, 2018). When informed that their care will be palliative, they need to adjust to this devastating information, complicated by a lack of understanding and trust and additionally managing both their physical and mental health symptoms (Jerwood et al., 2018).

Case study: Joe

Joe, 45, was diagnosed with schizophrenia in his 20s. He had regular 6-month health checks with his GP due to him taking clozapine. He had informed his GP for some time that he felt very tired and had difficulties with his bowel function, but this was attributed to his medication. He was admitted to hospital with bowel obstruction and was diagnosed with bowel cancer with lung metastases. He was informed that he only had months to live. He reluctantly agreed to go into a hospice but did not understand that his care was now palliative. During his stay, he became agitated, confused and distressed, and tried to leave on a number of occasions.

Activity 2.6   Critical thinking

* Why may Joe be feeling confused about his care?
* What would help Joe to understand his current situation?

There is an outline answer at the end of this chapter.

As discussed in Chapter 1 and illustrated above, people living with mental ill health frequently experience diagnostic overshadowing. This means that any physical symptoms they report are attributed to their mental health problem or medication rather than investigating whether there is an underlying physical health problem. Fatigue and lethargy are common symptoms for many people but can also be an indicator for cancer. Some of the medications used to treat mental ill health (see Chapter 7) do cause drowsiness and lethargy. It has been recognised that people who experience illnesses such as psychosis, schizophrenia and bipolar affective disorder are much more likely to die 15–20 years earlier than people without these conditions (Department of Health, 2014). This is due to a combination of reasons, such as the effects of the medication causing weight gain, dyslipidaemia and type 2 diabetes and additionally, poor diet and lack of exercise. They are also more likely to smoke cigarettes. All of these factors contribute to the development of CVD, which is the reason for the increased mortality. People who smoke are more likely to experience respiratory disease, in particular COPD. They may develop metabolic syndrome, which is a combination of diabetes, high blood pressure and obesity. To monitor their physical health they receive an annual physical check, including BMI, electrocardiogram and blood taken to check cholesterol and HbA1c (Naylor et al., 2016).

Holistic assessment

The culture of the Western world means that human experience is often thought about in a dichotomous fashion. Human behaviour is therefore thought to be either normal or abnormal. If a person is thought to be abnormal, the extremes of this position are pathological, either disordered or ill. In physical medicine this is helpful because if someone has a blood test which shows something out of the normal range, it gives the doctors clear clues about what might be going on. In mental health there are no blood tests which show normality or abnormality, so the conceptualisation of a problem is dependent upon the professional's experience and training and signs and symptoms (Sanders, 2019). A careful, thorough assessment is therefore crucial so that the professional can elicit as much information as possible to contribute to understanding and subsequent care planning.

George Engel (1913–1999) was an American psychiatrist and pioneer of the biopsychosocial model. This model of health considers the biological, psychological and social perspectives. The underlying assumption is that wellbeing comprises all these elements. Mental health nursing also favours this model and the nurse's assessment should therefore consider all these elements to be truly holistic. Engel advocated that nurses should ask not, what is wrong with you? but, what has happened? Reframing this simple question prompts the nurse to consider wider elements of the patient's presentation. Time and fear often prevent the nurse from wanting to ask such an open question. The patient's story is not just anecdotal, it is central to the development of their distress. Asking the patient what has led them here facilitates this story and at the same time offers the opportunity to build a rapport with the patient. This allows the nurse to think about how the patient's social situation has influenced their physical and psychological health. Activity 2.7 is designed to prompt you to consider a broad assessment of the patient's presentation.

Case study: Maggie

You are asked to make a home visit to Maggie, who is 57 years old and has failed to attend two recent appointments with the practice nurse to monitor her diabetes. The practice nurse is concerned as Maggie has suffered with depression in the past. When you get there Maggie is loath to let you in, saying that she is 'fine, thanks'. It is mid-afternoon, and she is in her dressing gown and has not brushed her hair, so you doubt that she is fine. As you look past her shoulder you can see her flat is chaotic and you can also see pizza boxes and insulin syringes on the floor. Maggie notices you looking at them and your recognition of her distress prompts her to let you in.

Activity 2.7   Critical thinking

- How are you going to approach Maggie? (Think about your manner and your verbal and non-verbal communication.)
- What might you want to know about Maggie's life and wellbeing? (Jot down some ideas in three bubbles: physical, mental, social.)
- How might you begin to help Maggie accept the help she so clearly needs?

There is an outline answer at the end of this chapter.

If the nurse does not consider Maggie's mental health as well as her diabetes, she would be likely to meet resistance to any interventions. The nurse needs to adopt a kind and gentle approach with Maggie, asking her what she can do which might be helpful. This gives Maggie a sense of control which will help facilitate some rapport. Once the nurse has made this connection with Maggie, she is then able to effectively assess Maggie's health, her emotional state and her social situation. At this point it might be helpful to start with some general conversation to build trust before moving on to a more specific question, such as asking why Maggie appears to have given up on herself. The nurse could try and establish whether Maggie is lonely and isolated because people who are lonely and isolated are nine times more likely to become sick (Maté, 2019). Is she fed up and miserable? Has something happened to her to make her abandon her diabetic regime? Although these questions are hard to ask, and you may feel intrusive, Maggie will get the sense that someone is listening to her story and caring about her. With the nurse's support and encouragement, Maggie is more likely to engage in the relationship and take control of her own recovery.

When you start nursing, asking personal questions of someone you don't know can feel strange. You are in a privileged position to be able to hear a person's most intimate worries and thoughts. As your course progresses and you develop more confidence, you will find this easier. Avoiding these personal questions means losing a wealth of information which could enable you to work more effectively with your patients by offering yourself with genuineness and honesty. Maggie will sense this and will then be likely to work with you on her recovery.

Nursing care and nursing skills in different settings

The last section of this chapter addresses the nursing care of individuals in different settings. Whether you are working as a student nurse in accident and emergency, older people's services, a medical ward or any mental health setting you could name, the fundamental skills you need to nurse anyone truly holistically are excellent communication skills. Being able to develop relationships with all kinds of people in any setting will enable you to assess the person's physical condition and emotional state concurrently.

Nurses from all fields must aim to work in a collaborative way with all their patients or service users. A degree of trust is necessary so that clients can share their difficulties with the nurse, set mutually determined goals, define the interventions designed to meet the goals and then review the plan together. To work in partnership, the nurse must first develop a rapport with the client so that they are engaged in their recovery as soon as possible.

Attachment theory suggests that early-life experiences with caregivers have a profound impact on the quality of relationships developed as an adult. Characteristic pattens of relating are formed which will influence every single relationship in later years. This includes how quickly we develop trust, how close we become to others and how dependent we are. Help-seeking behaviour is included in this (Green, 2010). For example, if a child repeatedly approaches their caregiver for security and is dismissed, ignored or on the receiving end of anger for bothering the adult, it is likely that the child will not readily seek help as an adult.

People display a variety of help-seeking behaviours, all of which are unique to the person and perfectly normal for them. Some people accept help readily, engage in their treatment and care and are easy to nurse. Other people do not always articulate their difficulties with clarity. Imagine for a moment that you are feeling ill but are struggling to get an appointment with the GP. It is hard to be assertive, and if you are unclear about the nature of your illness, i.e. if it is not a visible condition with clear signs and symptoms, it is even harder. Many people (arguably the older generation in particular) are quite stoic and may not readily ask for help, feeling that they should be tough enough to manage alone. Some people have had a difficult time with parents and may not trust you as a professional as a result. Many people have a strong need for personal control and will not necessarily be able to either recognise or acknowledge their anxiety or low mood, so you are going to need to develop skills to do this on their behalf. Anticipating and assessing someone's likely experience will make you the expert nurse you are aiming to be. It is a fine balance to aim for, so tread carefully and sensitively so you are not perceived as intrusive, or disempowering (Fisher, 2008). Pay attention to what the individual is saying (or not saying) so you can pick up any clues that the person is becoming guarded or irritated. If you are in doubt about the person's experience, ask them. If someone is struggling to articulate their experience, wait. Building a healing relationship takes time. Assessing the illness, the pain, the fear, anxiety or any other stressful emotion will enable you to help the person work through any denial and access the help and support needed. Being present with any distress provides comfort and maximises the chances of the person participating and taking control of their situation and their recovery. Many nurses believe that they are most effective when they are doing something for a patient. It is however an essential skill to be able to 'just be' with a patient (Benner, 1984).

Chapter summary

This chapter has explored why it is important to recognise the relationship between physical and mental health and the importance of ensuring that you always provide holistic assessment and care. The chapter has discussed how specific physical conditions affect a person's mental health and how people living with mental ill health may also develop physical illnesses. The activities and case studies illustrate how you can recognise, assess and care for people.

Activities: Brief outline answers

Activity 2.2 Reflection (page 26)

When we are unwell, we initially may be anxious regarding the cause, the length of the illness and the impact on our employment, family and caring role as we may be unable to maintain our normal activities. Therefore, it can affect other people in our family who need to take on additional roles. Also we may be fearful of what this illness indicates, especially if there were unusual symptoms.

Activity 2.3 Critical thinking (page 30)

John may be reluctant to seek help for his symptoms as he is fearful of what he may be told. He is frightened that he has the same condition as his brother and that his death is imminent. John tends to use a maladaptive coping strategy and avoids visiting his GP as he hopes his symptoms will resolve. If he does not seek help his symptoms may worsen and he may also experience a myocardial infarction like his brother, or a stroke. If he visited the GP earlier, he could have a full assessment, which would determine an underlying cause and he would be able to start treatment if required. Using alcohol to manage his symptoms can cause additional health problems such as alcohol dependence, so he will gradually increase his drinking to have the same effect and may become both physically and psychologically dependent. Alcohol has detrimental effects on all systems of the body, particularly the GI and nervous system.

Activity 2.4 Critical thinking (page 31)

Joan may be anxious as she is fearful of not being able to breathe and therefore of dying. As she becomes more anxious this will exacerbate her breathlessness and therefore her anxiety will increase further. Sarah's intervention was helpful as it provided comfort and compassion to Joan but also the reassurance of help and support.

Activity 2.5 Critical thinking (page 33)

Your concerns would be that Faith may be at risk of or is experiencing symptoms of an eating disorder such as anorexia nervosa. Avoiding food will worsen her symptoms of Crohn's disease and lead to severe malnutrition and Faith could become severely unwell.

Julie needs to sensitively ask Faith about her eating patterns and how she feels about her body image. She should discuss with her about the risks of her stopping eating and the impact on her body. More importantly, she should listen to Faith's concerns and support her, arranging to see her again within 2 weeks to review her. If her symptoms persist and she has not gained weight or is losing more weight, she may require referral to the mental health team.

Activity 2.6 Critical thinking (page 34)

Joe will be confused as he does not clearly understand what is happening and why he is not receiving care for his cancer, particularly as he had informed his GP he was unwell and his symptoms were not investigated. So, he is simultaneously having to accept the news that he has cancer and that he is dying. Also, when receiving traumatic information we do not recall everything that has been said and can misinterpret information. This can lead to confusion and misunderstanding.

It would be beneficial for Joe to meet with his health care team to discuss what is happening as often as required and for him to be given the time and space to understand and ask questions. It may be helpful for a friend or partner to be with him when these meetings occur so he can discuss this afterwards.

Activity 2.7 Critical thinking (page 36)

There are no right or wrong answers to this case study. A few prompts are given here to show you the broad remit of the information you may decide to elicit.

Maggie is presenting as unhappy and unmotivated. If you try and mirror Maggie's energy levels, and moderate your voice to match hers, you will not come across as too loud or excitable. This will help you establish some connection with her. Keep an open posture and maintain good eye contact. Consider Maggie's personal space because she is cautious about having a visitor. Show her your ID and let her know that it was the practice nurse who asked you to visit due to her missed appointments. This demonstrates your honesty and provides a rationale for your visit which will help to build some trust.

Physical

You will want to know how long she has been diagnosed with diabetes and how long she has managed the blood tests herself, as this gives you a clue about what you could expect her to manage when she is feeling better. You will want to know more about her blood tests, how often she normally does them, what her usual results are and when they were last done. You might encourage her to put her used sharps in a sharps box so that she keeps herself safe. You might also ask her about her usual diet, and gently question why she has needed to order pizzas frequently.

Mental

You might want to ask Maggie what her mood is like. How often is she still in her dressing gown by mid-afternoon? Is there a reason for this? Has she been unwell? Did she sleep badly or has this been going on for some time? How does she normally sleep? Is she too unmotivated to cook anything healthy?

Social

Does she have any relationships in her life? Partner, children, friends? Has she fallen out with someone?

What does she do all day? Does she work? If so, is there a problem at work? What activities does she enjoy?

Has something happened which has knocked her mood? (It may be worth asking directly about her housing and benefit status.)

Maggie needs to accept some help but appears loath to acknowledge this.

If you offer to help her with whatever she prefers, she then sets the goals. She may want help to do her hair or pick up some shopping. It is worth investing in this, so that your relationship is paramount. If you focus upon encouraging her to resume her bloods or take anti-depressants you are likely to jeopardise the relationship and are then at risk of alienating her further.

Further reading

De Vries, J and Timmins, F (2017) *Understanding Psychology for Nursing Students.* London: SAGE.

This book demonstrates how psychology applies to nursing.

Useful website

http://dwed.org.uk/

Diabetics with Eating Disorders (DWED) is a charity organisation that supports and advocates for people with both type 1 diabetes and an eating disorder.

Chapter 3 Understanding mental health problems

Steve Trenoweth

NMC Future Nurse: Standards of Proficiency for Registered Nurses

This chapter will address the following platforms and proficiencies:

Platform 1: Being an accountable professional

At the point of registration, the registered nurse will be able to:

1.9   understand the need to base all decisions regarding care and interventions on people's needs and preferences, recognising and addressing any personal and external factors that may unduly influence their decisions.

Platform 2: Promoting health and preventing ill health

At the point of registration, the registered nurse will be able to:

2.5   promote and improve mental, physical, behavioural and other health related outcomes by understanding and explaining the principles, practice and evidence-base for health screening programmes.

Platform 3: Assessing needs and planning care

At the point of registration, the registered nurse will be able to:

3.2   demonstrate and apply knowledge of body systems and homeostasis, human anatomy and physiology, biology, genomics, pharmacology and social and behavioural sciences when undertaking full and accurate person-centred nursing assessments and developing appropriate care plans.

(Continued)

(Continued)

3.3 demonstrate and apply knowledge of all commonly encountered mental, physical, behavioural and cognitive health conditions, medication usage and treatments when undertaking full and accurate assessments of nursing care needs and when developing, prioritising and reviewing person-centred care plans.

3.5 demonstrate the ability to accurately process all information gathered during the assessment process to identify needs for individualised nursing care and develop person-centred evidence-based plans for nursing interventions with agreed goals.

Platform 4: Providing and evaluating care

At the point of registration, the registered nurse will be able to:

4.4 demonstrate the knowledge and skills required to support people with commonly encountered mental health, behavioural, cognitive and learning challenges, and act as a role model for others in providing high quality nursing interventions to meet people's needs.

Platform 7: Coordinating care

At the point of registration, the registered nurse will be able to:

7.5 understand and recognise the need to respond to the challenges of providing safe, effective and person-centred nursing care for people who have co-morbidities and complex care needs.

Chapter aims

After reading this chapter, you will be able to:

- understand the different meanings of mental ill health;
- understand the various theories and models of mental health and ill health;
- explain how a holistic viewpoint can aid all nurses with helping people to improve their mental health.

Introduction

In this chapter we will explore the different meanings of mental ill health. We will then explore the various theories and models of mental health and ill health, before looking at the complex relationship between them all, and how a holistic viewpoint can help all nurses to support people with improving their mental health.

Clarifying terminology

The words that we use in our lives can be a subtle way of communicating perceptions and biases. Words can act as symbols for a larger set of, often otherwise unstated, assumptions and ideas. Look at the example given in the case study below.

Case study: Sandra

Sandra has a long history of hearing voices, which has had a devastating effect on her life. She is often very angry with mental health services and sometimes she breaks off contact with them, as she feels they do not always meet her needs. Sandra has been hospitalised in a mental health facility against her will six times in the last 4 years. However, when she feels well, Sandra manages to do some voluntary work in a local Age Concern charity shop. Recently, things have been difficult for Sandra as she struggles with the break-up of a long-term relationship.

Sandra has been diagnosed with diabetes and is being seen by a diabetic nurse specialist with whom she recently had an argument. Sandra felt that the nurse specialist 'kept going on' about her diagnosis of schizophrenia, which Sandra feels has nothing to do with her diabetes. Sandra is also under the care of a community mental health nurse, with whom she generally has a good relationship. Sandra relates the argument she had with the diabetic nurse specialist:

She kept telling me I am mentally ill. She said, 'Because you are mentally ill you need to remember to take your diabetes medication'. I found her patronising and I asked her what she meant by my being mentally ill. She thought I was stupid. I asked if she was mentally healthy. I don't know what good mental health is and she didn't seem to know either.

In this case study, Sandra asked what seem to be straightforward questions – what do you mean by mental illness? what is mental health? The concepts of *mental health* and *mental illness* are terms which are value-laden – that is, they are imbued with more meaning than can be found by a dictionary definition. Such terms carry with them a set of personal, social and cultural assumptions. Sandra, for example, felt that the nurse specialist saw her as 'stupid' because of her mental health issue.

Activity 3.1   Reflection

Think for a moment and jot down any words you associate with the term *schizophrenia*.

- What does the term imply to you?
- How did you develop your ideas about the term? That is, where do you get your ideas from?

There is an outline answer at the end of this chapter.

You might have thought that the term schizophrenia was a *mental illness* or a *psychiatric diagnosis*. You might have even jotted down the term *madness*. You might have assumed that people with this diagnosis are dangerous or violent, or that they need long-term institutional care.

In this book we tend to use terms such as *mental health problems, mental ill health* or *mental distress* to encompass the broad experience of all people with psychological difficulties rather than words which are medically bound, such as *mental illness* or *mental disorder,* which may convey or reinforce the view that mental health problems have a biological or psychiatric origin. As we shall see later, there are indeed many different interpretations of mental health and mental distress.

It can be quite difficult to reflect on where our ideas, values and assumptions come from. Often, they are transmitted by our parents, friends and siblings. Sometimes the media (books, magazines, newspapers as well as film and television) represents and reinforces a particular view about groups of people. We may be unaware that the use of our terms may cause offence. While such symbols can give people a sense of common identity, they can also lead to stigma and stereotyping, which can often go unchallenged. In nursing care, it is vital that we are aware of such symbols and that our culturally imbued and socially constructed knowledge does not affect the quality of care that we provide.

For example, we must not assume that an individual's problems centre solely on a medical diagnosis. This is called *diagnostic overshadowing*, where one diagnosis or condition is given pre-eminence over other health issues that an individual may be experiencing. Take, for example, a person who has been diagnosed with, and is receiving treatment for, cancer. This is very likely to be a time of considerable stress and distress for the individual and friends and family. However, the attention of nursing and other health care staff may be focused on treating the cancer and may not recognise or respond to psychological distress that may be experienced. As such, nurses must recognise that anyone can experience mental distress, regardless of whether or not they have a diagnosed mental illness, and it is the duty of the nurse to respond to the overall needs of their patients, including psychological support.

What is mental illness?

In Chapter 1, we explored the concept of mental health, which reflects our ability to cope with life stress and work productively and make a contribution to our communities (World Health Organization, 2018). We explored the idea that mental health is something which we personally sense and feel when we see ourselves behaving in mentally healthy ways. So, what might *mental illness* refer to?

Activity 3.2 Reflection

The use of the term 'illness' when describing mental health problems carries with it many implications. Take a few moments to think about and note down what is generally implied by the term 'illness'.

There is an outline answer at the end of the chapter.

You might have noted that an 'illness' is a disease arising from a germ or infection, or some physiological problem within the body. If so, you might argue that an illness implies a medical or biological problem associated with some form of bodily dysfunction. Now if we were to apply this to the concept of *mental illness* we might assume that mental health problems have a biological basis arising from some form of anatomical defect or physiological dysfunction within the brain.

When we talk of a mental 'illness' we are, technically, talking of a mental health problem that has been assigned a psychiatric diagnosis (psychiatry is the branch of medicine which diagnoses and treats mental disorders). There are two main medical diagnosis systems (or taxonomies) which are currently in use: the World Health Organization's *International Classification of Diseases for Mortality and Morbidity Statistics* (11th revision) (ICD-11: World Health Organization, 2019) and the American Psychiatric Association's *Diagnostic and Statistical Manual of Mental Disorders* (5th ed.) (DSM-V: American Psychiatric Association, 2013). Both of these systems attempt to catalogue mental disorders by assigning a diagnosis based on an assessment of symptom clusters. For example, if one is experiencing unpredictable attacks of severe anxiety with sudden onset of palpitations, chest pain, choking sensations, dizziness and feelings of unreality, with fear of dying, losing control or going mad, then a diagnosis, using the ICD-11 classification of *panic disorder* may be warranted, such as is the case with Leah in the case study below.

Case study: Leah

Leah is a 28-year-old housewife and formerly a registered adult nurse. She spent many years working with sick people and specialised in intensive care. She is very proud of her nursing career and feels that she made an important contribution to people's lives.

Leah is an articulate, intelligent woman who feels ashamed of her inability to cope. Leah has a child of 5 years and says that her panic attacks started soon after he was born. Leah is constantly worried, very anxious and unable to cope with looking after her child. When she has a panic

(Continued)

(Continued)

attack she starts to tremble, her pulse races, she has chest pain and she feels dizzy and sick. The frequency and intensity of her panic attacks have been increasing recently to the point where they have become severe and disabling, leading to a functional impairment in her everyday life.

She says that things are out of control for her and she is at the mercy of her panic attacks. She says she feels she is a hopeless mother and that nothing she ever does is right. Her husband wants another child but she doesn't know how she is going to cope. She doesn't know what to do when she is in this state. She tries to keep it hidden from her husband, who says she is just being 'silly'.

In this case study, we can see that Leah is experiencing many of the key features of a *panic disorder* as defined by the ICD-11, namely anxiety, worry, feelings of being unable to cope and that things are out of control, experience of chest pain and dizziness.

There is evidence which, seemingly, links underlying biological dysfunction of the central nervous system with mental health problems. For example, chronic and enduring depression and stress and post-traumatic stress disorder can lead to damage of the brain, particularly the hippocampus, amygdala and frontal cortex (Perna et al., 2003). A depressive disorder may result from physical trauma to the brain where the ability of the brain to transmit information is disrupted (Brown, 2006). Some degenerative brain diseases such as Alzheimer's have clear organic aetiologies; for example, neuroimaging seems to indicate that people with Alzheimer's have neural tangles in their brain which appear to kill brain cells. Poor nutrition and diet have also been linked to mental health problems (Mental Health Foundation, 2006). For example, some nutrients such as folic acid, omega-3 fatty acids, selenium and tryptophan appear to reduce the symptoms of depression. Some infections which can affect the development of the fetus, such as prenatal influenza, can increase the risk of a diagnosis of schizophrenia in adulthood (Brown, 2006). There also appears to be heritability factors associated with many mental illnesses (Kring and Johnson, 2019). Studies which attempt to capture the role of heredity typically explore the incidence of illnesses in families and amongst twins, assuming that if identical twins raised apart have similar rates, then this would suggest a genetic predisposition or vulnerability towards a particular disorder. For example, some twin studies suggest that identical twins are three times more likely to develop schizophrenia if their twin also has this diagnosis than non-identical twins (Kring and Johnson, 2019).

Activity 3.3   Reflection

If you believe that mental distress has a biological origin and is thus symptomatic of psychiatric dysfunction and disorder, what sorts of treatments do you think might be offered?

There is an outline answer at the end of the chapter.

The (bio)medical model

Look back at your notes from Activities 3.2 and 3.3. If you feel that mental health problems have a biological origin, then you are likely to suggest a biological response, such as the prescription of psychiatric medication. The medical model claims that biological factors (such as the anatomy and physiology of an individual's nervous system and their genetic make-up) are crucial risk factors in the development of a mental illness (Engel, 1977). For example, an excess of the neurotransmitter *dopamine* has been linked to schizophrenia. Indeed, if one perceives that the root cause of a mental health problem is physical, then treatment which is prescribed is likely to be targeted at a biological level, and as such the management of symptoms is likely to involve medical interventions, such as the prescription of medication, electroconvulsive therapy (ECT) or, in extreme cases, psychosurgery.

There are, however, some people who dispute that mental distress is an 'illness' or suggest that the role of biological predeterminants of mental distress has been over-emphasised. Assuming for a moment that there is clear agreement between people in terms of the diagnosis of a person's mental illness (Bentall (2003) suggests that there is not), there is as yet no clear evidence to prove the connection between biological dysfunction and mental health problems. The interpretation of twin studies, for example, is not always clear, with some suggestions that findings of studies are based on a poor statistical analysis of results (Bentall, 2003), and there are few studies of twins being raised fully apart to provide conclusive evidence (Kring and Johnson, 2019).

Engel (1977) argued that the biomedical model may restrict our understanding of health and illness in that it does not help us to understand how beliefs, expectations and hopes impact on the trajectory of health and illness. For example, when arriving at a psychiatric diagnosis the psychiatrist seeks to make 'objective' judgements about a person's mental state and capacity. There is, of course, a danger of seeing a person solely in terms of their diagnosis – this process is known as *labelling*. As we saw with Leah, once such a label has been applied it can overshadow other aspects of the person until the person is only seen in terms of the diagnosis.

In fairness, however, people who subscribe to the biomedical model do not inevitably rule out the interaction of biological factors with, for example, environmental experiences of an individual. Geneticists, for example, might argue that an individual has a *predisposition* to a particular illness but that environmental factors play an important role in whether this gene finds expression. Unquestionably, the medical model has offered much to people who experience mental distress and has helped many on their road to recovery, and we would be unwise to dismiss this approach. However, we must also remember that the medical model is just one approach and that people experiencing mental distress should have available to them a range of options they can choose from to help them meet their particular needs and wishes.

Sociological theories of mental ill health

There are many interpretations of mental ill health in terms of its origins (*aetiology*) and many forms of possible treatment. Perceptions of mental distress have changed over time, not only in terms of its aetiology but also in terms of how subsequently it is thought best to help.

In Activities 3.2 and 3.3, you explored the concept of illness and how biological understandings of illness might lead to medical treatment. In the next activity, you are asked to consider alternative views of mental ill health:

Activity 3.4 Points to consider

1. How might different peoples or cultures see mental ill health differently?
2. How might societies' views of mental health and illness lead to the development of services?
3. What alternative explanations are there to account for mental ill health?

For each alternative explanation, try to think of how alternative explanations might lead to alternative treatments for mental health issues.

There is an outline answer at the end of the chapter.

In answering the first question of Activity 3.4 you might have said, thinking back to the idea of symbolic interactionism, that people and cultures 'construct' meanings surrounding health and illness and that some cultures have a scientific interpretation of health and illness whilst others rely on spiritual or lay beliefs regarding aetiology and treatment of ailments. For example, one culture may interpret a vision of Christ as a miracle; another may see this as a visual hallucination and a symptom of psychosis.

Sociological models

Social, sociocultural and interpersonal models argue that the basis of mental distress is grounded in the social world. This approach assumes that the way people feel and think is affected by the circumstances in which they live and work, which are in turn the product of economic and sociopolitical conditions in society (Rogers and Pilgrim, 2021). For example, social stressors arising from job loss and unemployment, loss of a close friend, relative or spouse, stress from within the family, chronic social adversity (for example, poverty), stigma, social exclusion and a lack of community acceptance and tolerance, lack of social support and isolation and a lack of a sense of belonging in a community can have a profound influence on our mental health (Holmes and Rahe, 1967; Bentall, 2003; Rogers and Pilgrim, 2021).

Sociological understandings of mental health and ill health stress the importance of considering the impact of socioeconomic inequalities and disadvantageous life situations, stigma, social exclusion and the impact of psychiatric services on individuals with protected characteristics (such as race, religion and sexual orientation) (Nazroo and Iley, 2011; Rogers and Pilgrim, 2021). Such understandings stress that individuals may have different interpretations of their own health and illness, which may be influenced by their own personal cultural experiences, and it is important to clarify this as it may be a barrier to nursing and health care in general. For example, lay theories of mental health may be at odds with views held by health professionals and with known scientific 'best available evidence'. Individuals may also hold unrealistic expectations with regard to achieving maximal physical or mental health. Therefore, in answer to the third question in Activity 3.4, you may have argued that modern mental health services in the UK are predominantly medical and scientific in their outlook. It is fair to say that the medical approach is seemingly the predominant paradigm, but this belies the fact that there are many different interpretations, models and theories of mental distress. In answering the first question, you might have, quite correctly, thought that there are psychological and social factors which underpin mental health issues. It is to these alternative models of mental ill health that we now turn.

Indeed, there is much evidence that social inequalities and social disadvantage are disabling and are risk factors which are likely to increase mental distress and/or contribute to relapse amongst those who already experience mental distress. For example, people who have been abused or who are the victims of domestic violence have higher rates of mental health problems. Prisoners in overcrowded environments have a high rate of mental health problems, such as suicide and self-harm (Howard League for Penal Reform, 2016). People with an identified mental health problem are more likely to be excluded from work; those with a common mental disorder are four to five times more likely to be unemployed, twice as likely to be on income support and four to five times more likely to be getting invalidity benefits compared to the general population; financial pressures are the most frequently cited cause of a depressive disorder; people with mental health problems are more likely to be in debt, to be trapped in poverty and have difficulties managing money than other members of the general population.

For Harry Stack Sullivan (1953), mental health problems were reflective of social 'problems of living'. Durkheim's *Suicide: A Study in Sociology*, published in 1897, argued that suicide was a reflection of the degree of social integration that an individual experienced. Higher rates, he suggested, occurred when people were insufficiently integrated into social groups. Brown and Harris' seminal 1978 work *The Social Origins of Depression* argued that loss and the stresses and strains in women's daily experiences are implicated in depression. For example, ongoing, stressful social and interpersonal circumstances, such as longstanding difficulty in relationships, can lead to an increased likelihood of their developing a depressive disorder. Such vulnerability in women, Brown and Harris found, may be enhanced by having three children under the age of 14 years, not working outside the home, having no one to confide in and loss of one's mother by death or separation before the age of 11 years. For people with a mental health problem, their psychiatric diagnoses may be more than a way of classifying mental disorder. Some would argue that they add to the 'problems of living' of this group by acting as a label by which people are stigmatised, thereby reinforcing, perpetuating and even possibly justifying social disadvantage.

There are also wide cultural variations in the interpretation and perceptions of health and illness. In mental health, we can see this in cross-cultural research into depression and anxiety. For example, when presenting initially with depression, Latin American people tend to report more bodily symptoms whereas people in the USA and Western Europe have higher rates of reported headaches (Morrison and Bennett, 2006). There are also gender differences in the perceptions and interpretations of mental and physical health and illness. For example, men have a shorter lifespan, higher rates of physical health problems and engage in more risk-taking behaviours which have a health impact (such as smoking, unprotected sex, unprotected exposure to the sun, and so on) and higher incidences of drug/alcohol use and suicide. Such health issues, it has been argued, are influenced by, and often seem to reflect, socialisation into particular gender roles where the male role may be culturally imbued with assumptions of social obligations and the apparent need to be strong, achievement-oriented and competitive. That is, it seems that there are barriers. Goldberg (1977) called this the 'bind' of masculinity and being a man, statistically at least, may seriously damage your physical health and mental wellbeing.

What is considered to be 'good' mental health and mental ill health, and the cultural presentation of symptoms of mental ill health, are therefore relative judgements and definitions of what is mentally healthy can change across time, across cultures and between individuals based on socialisation and one's own personal experience. Sometimes, of course, the opinions of others about our mental health may differ from our own personal judgements.

Psychological models

Broadly, the various psychological models and theories suggest that mental distress is underpinned by how one thinks and feels about oneself and the world and/or how one behaves. This in turn has an impact on how we feel about ourselves (such as our self-esteem, self-confidence, and so on), and our confidence and our place in the world.

Behavioural models argue that we learn (or are 'conditioned') by our environment. *Behaviourism* is a branch of psychology which assumes that the behaviour of an organism may be changed (or 'conditioned') by environmental events (or 'stimuli'). There are two main theories: *classical conditioning* and *operant conditioning*. We acquire much of our learning through classical conditioning. For example, if you are hungry and smell your favourite food, you are likely to salivate. This was the basis of a study by Ivan

Pavlov in the early 20th century. Every time food was presented to a dog, a bell was struck. Over time, the dog would salivate when the bell was struck *before* the presentation of the food. It had learned to *associate* the sound of the bell with the presentation of the food. Classical conditioning is thought to be a mechanism by which people acquire phobias and is based on work undertaken by Watson and Rayner in 1920. Here is how it is thought to work: a person may be exposed to a frightening situation (such as a loud noise, or a disturbing event which leads to a fear response) at the same time as experiencing a neutral stimulus (this is an object or event that would otherwise be non-threatening – the smell of coffee, for example). This neutral stimulus, then, may become associated with the fearful situation. Over time fear is experienced on presentation of the neutral stimulus – the person has been conditioned to respond fearfully to the neutral stimulus.

Operant conditioning sees an important relationship between an action and its consequences – called the law of effect. This law suggests that an action which has good consequences will tend to be repeated, whereas if an action has bad consequences it will tend not to be repeated. The stronger the association between a stimulus and a positive effect (that is, the strength of *positive reinforcement*), the more likely that the stimulus will condition one's behaviour.

Skinner suggested that our response to a stimulus tends to persist and will survive even if, occasionally, it produces an unfavourable response. In addition to positive reinforcement (where favourable consequences are likely to strengthen an association between a stimulus and a response), Skinner also suggested that *negative reinforcement* (where a favourable response is associated with the termination of an unpleasant stimulus) is also likely to increase the frequency of a response. For example, one may learn to associate not opening a utility bill, which requires us to part with money we don't have, with temporary peace of mind. One may think, 'I don't have to worry about something I don't know about'. Similarly, not studying for an exam helps us to deal with exam anxiety. We ignore and avoid the reality of the exam! Both of these events help us to cope, but only in a short-term way. They are ultimately *maladaptive* and do not help us to cope in a positive way. The short-term relief of an unpleasant stimulus can lead to long-term consequences. Not studying for an exam may be tension relieving but it will not help you to pass it. How might you condition yourself to develop more *adaptive* responses to exam anxiety? That is, how can you learn to associate exam revision with positive consequences?

Another historically very important psychological theory which seeks to account for mental distress is that of psychodynamic theory, stemming from the work of Sigmund Freud. It is not possible for us to give a comprehensive overview of his complex theory (of which there have been many subsequent modifications made by later psychoanalysts). However, the essence of the theory states that mental distress is grounded in our early development. Problems which have not been satisfactorily resolved during our development may find expression in later life.

The recovery approach

As we saw in Chapter 1, the *recovery approach* has been influential in mental health services in England. It is a person-centred approach which comes directly from the service user movement. The recovery approach attaches importance to the service users' experience of the process of empowerment that leads to more fulfilling and meaningful lives rather than to what services do *for* people, often in response to crisis (National Institute for Mental Health in England (NIMHE), 2005).

The recovery approach also draws a distinction between *complete recovery* (in which an individual returns to their prior level of functioning, implying that the person has been 'cured' or *recovered*) and *social recovery* (which focuses on helping the person *towards* recovery, and involves an emphasis on social support, realistic planning, significant working relationships, encouragement, appropriate treatment, choice and self-management) (Warner, 1985; Matthews, 2008; Trenoweth et al., 2017). In the latter case, much emphasis is placed on the ongoing process of *recovering* from mental health challenges. Hence, recovery in this sense:

> *is not about regaining a problem-free life – whose life is? It is about living life more resourcefully, living a satisfying and contributing life, in spite of limitations caused by a continuing vulnerability to disabling distress* (Watkins, 2001, page 45).

More contemporary perspectives of the recovery approach in England have been influenced by a guiding statement published in 2005 by the now defunct National Institute for Mental Health in England (NIMHE) (Figure 3.1).

A broad vision of recovery [...] involves a process of changing one's orientation and behaviour from a negative focus on a troubling event, condition or circumstance to the positive restoration, rebuilding, reclaiming or taking control of one's life. Furthermore, a recovery-oriented system of care will:

- Focus on people rather than services.
- Monitor outcomes rather than performance.
- Emphasise strengths rather than deficits or dysfunction.
- Educate people who provide services, schools, employers, the media and the public to combat stigma.
- Foster collaboration between those who need support and those who support them as an alternative to coercion.
- Through enabling and supporting self-management, promote autonomy and, as a result, decrease the need for people to rely on formal service and professional supports.

Figure 3.1 Guiding statement on recovery (National Institute for Mental Health in England (NIMHE), 2005).

In 2008, the Centre for Mental Health published an influential and important document entitled *Making Recovery a Reality* (Shepherd et al., 2008). It provided indicators of how recovery can be promoted through practice in mental health settings, recognising the importance of a home, employment, a living wage and genuine control over their life. It reinforced the need for services to be orientated towards hope and emphasised the need to build on an individual's strengths and abilities in the process of their recovery.

In July 2009, the Future Vision Coalition (a group of UK-based charities and mental health organisations) set out a new vision for mental health. It argues for a broader public health approach and sees that good mental health is important for an overall good quality of life. In this sense, mental health is an issue for everyone in society. It argues for effective positive mental health promotion to be a policy priority for the UK Government, including building resilience and targeted prevention work with 'at-risk' groups and individuals and in areas such as prisons, schools and in workplaces. As Martin Seligman (2002, page xi) put it, people *want more than just to correct their weaknesses*, hoping to live a life imbued with personal meaning and happiness. In this sense, Seligman (2002) argues that happiness is not the hedonism of momentary pleasures but 'authentic' and enduring happiness where one recognises and plays to one's signature strengths. Typically, in helping people to find such happiness, the starting point is not on deficits but on strengths, such as wisdom and knowledge; courage; humanity and love; positive relationships with communities; temperance; and transcendence (strengths which help to connect people to something larger than themselves, such as aesthetic appreciation, a sense of purpose and spirituality) (Seligman, 2002). For Seligman (2008, page 15), the focus on positive health *is not only desirable in its own right ... it is likely to be a buffer against physical and mental illness.*

Mental ill health as a complex phenomenon

Mental ill health is a complex phenomenon and as such it is not likely that any one approach will account for the various dimensions of an individual's experience. As our knowledge and understanding of mental health and mental ill health increase, there will inevitably be a rethink about how the various parts of the jigsaw fit together. As such, there will continue to be a need for various diverse theories and models which seek to account for an individual's experience (and extensions or revisions to existing ones) and a variety of interventions that individuals may wish to draw upon to support their recovery.

In this sense, there is no 'correct' model or one theory which can stand as 'truth' when we attempt to understand the totality of an individual's experience of mental distress (Engel, 1977). In fact, each of the models and approaches explored here focuses on different aspects of human functioning and helps us to understand different aspects of experience. Potentially, therefore, the models and theories are *complementary* and taken together can develop our understanding of an individual's distress and likewise open up many different and varied avenues of care and treatment. This point was stressed by Engel in 1977 when he proposed a *biopsychosocial* model of disease. Here Engel argued that a purely biomedical approach to mental distress was limiting and that there is a need to explore how psychological and social factors combined with the biological to affect the trajectory of illnesses. Here, Engel (1977) was arguing that there is a need to include the *person* as well as the illness in developing an understanding of their health problems. Likewise, also in 1977, Zubin and Spring were arguing for a *new view of schizophrenia* which sought to explore how stressors could lead to a breakdown of coping in people vulnerable to schizophrenia. They assumed that people have a degree of vulnerability to schizophrenia which is *inborn* (for example, genetic and the 'internal environment' of the individual) and *acquired* (for example, the influence of traumas, perinatal complications and life events) which due to the interaction and presence of certain circumstances will challenge and provoke a crisis for a person's mental health. Such challenging circumstances (or 'exogenous stressors'), Zubin and Spring (1977) argue, include life event stresses (such as bereavement, marriage, divorce) which require a degree of coping and readjustment in the person's life. In vulnerable people, there may be a failure to cope and adapt to such stresses, which may place their mental health under strain and increase the likelihood of mental ill health or relapse.

It might be tempting to think of *mental ill health* or *mental illness* as the exact polar opposite of *mental health*. That is, that one either 'has' mental health or mental illness as if they were discrete categories to which one is assigned. However, it is more fitting to see mental health and mental illness as existing on a continuum and as such one may experience *degrees* of mental health (and mental distress) and this varies and fluctuates at various times in our lives. One of the ways in which our mental health may fluctuate might be as a response to the amount of stress that we experience in our lives. Indeed, it seems that we as individuals can vary in response to exposure to stress, as Zubin and Spring (1977) suggested above. In this sense there is no 'us' and 'them'. There are not 'mentally ill people' as a distinct or separate group but all of 'us' who can, and do, experience varying degrees of mental health and mental distress.

A holistic view of mental health

A more holistic view sees mental health as encompassing not only such social factors, but also physical, psychological, emotional and spiritual dimensions of self. As such, the model is an attempt to *pool the wisdom from all of the models* (Zubin and Spring, 1977, page 109). A holistic model has five interconnected dimensions (Swinton, 2001):

1. physical (the biological aspect of our selves);

2. social (our relationships with others);

3. emotional (the way in which we feel about ourselves and our lives);

4. psychological (beliefs and perceptions that we hold about ourselves and others);

5. spiritual (the meaning that we attach to our lives).

Swinton's model suggests that our experience of health, and ill health, is likely to be multidimensional rather than one-dimensional. Importantly, as one dimension is affected this will impact on the other dimension of ourselves. This suggests that our physical and mental wellbeing are interrelated. For example, a problem with our physical health is likely to have implications for our social, emotional, psychological and spiritual wellbeing.

Chapter summary

In this chapter we have looked at how terminology can affect our perceptions – and in particular our understandings of mental health problems. We have discussed how mental health and mental ill health may exist on a continuum and as such one may experience *degrees* of mental health (and mental distress) and that this varies and fluctuates at various times in our lives. We have also explored the models and theories which have sought to account for mental distress (including the medical, psychological, social and positive health/recovery approach). We have also explored a unifying framework for understanding the person, namely that of holism, as a way of appreciating the totality of the person's experience, including their mental and physical dimension of self, which may be of assistance to all nurses in discharging their professional duty of providing holistic care.

Activities: Brief outline answers

Activity 3.1 Reflection (page 43)

The term schizophrenia is technically a medical diagnosis which refers to a set of experiences where a person may experience delusions or hallucinations. It is often used incorrectly to imply a split personality. You may have been exposed to media representations of people diagnosed with schizophrenia and sometimes attention-grabbing headlines. Nurses must be able to challenge this 'received wisdom' as it might have significant implications for care.

Activity 3.2 Reflection (page 45)

Illness is poor health resulting from disease – a state of being sick. Other words associated with the term can include sickness, impairment, disorder, ailment, affliction, and so forth.

The World Health Organization defines mental health as:

> a state of well-being in which an individual realizes his or her own abilities, can cope with the normal stresses of life, can work productively and is able to make a contribution to his or her community. In this positive sense, mental health is the foundation for individual well-being and the effective functioning of a community (World Health Organization, 1946).

In this sense mental health represents our ability to cope with, function in and be a part of our communities.

Activity 3.3 Reflection (page 46)

People who see a biological basis for mental disorder would most commonly prescribe a medical treatment such as medication, ECT or, in extreme cases, psychosurgery.

Activity 3.4 Points to consider (page 48)

Constructions of mental health and mental ill health are often socially determined and this changes over time. In fact, whether or not something is even considered to be a mental health issue is subject to change. Sometimes, cultures have alternative ways of viewing what we might perceive to be mental ill health, and their understandings may have supernatural or religious bases. It is clear that if a society believes in the medical basis for mental ill health then it will fund medical services as a response. If it sees mental ill health in supernatural terms, such hospitals would be irrelevant and alternative help and advice may be sought. In addition to the medical approach, there are psychological and social models which seek to explain mental ill health.

Further reading

Bentall, R (2003) *Madness Explained: Psychosis and Human Nature.* London: Penguin.

An important book, if rather complex at times, which argues against the medical understanding of mental ill health. Bentall argues that mental illness labels such as schizophrenia are meaningless and criticises the medical approach to mental health care.

Glossary

Adaptive	Helpful responses/good coping
Aetiology	The origins or causes of an illness or health issue
Behaviourism	A learning theory which suggests that human behaviour results from conditioning
Biopsychosocial model	A model which examines the biological, psychological and social aspects of health and illness
Classical conditioning	Stemming from the work of Ivan Pavlov, in this form of learning a neutral stimulus becomes associated with another stimulus to produce a similar response
Complete recovery	A cure for an illness or disorder; complete abatement of symptoms
Labelling	In sociology, this is the process of describing a person to identify aberrant behaviour
Maladaptive	Unhelpful responses/poor coping
Negative automatic thoughts	Negative thinking about self, the world or the future which occurs to a person seemingly without prior thought
Negative reinforcement	Removal of an unpleasant stimulus to increase the occurrence of a behaviour
Operant conditioning	A form of conditioning where the reinforcement of a behaviour influences its occurrence
Positive reinforcement	Reward for a behaviour which increases its occurrence
Social recovery	A return to effective social functioning

Table 3.1   Glossary

Chapter 4

Legal and ethical frameworks in mental health care

Tula Brannelly and Josie Tuck

NMC Future Nurse: Standards of Proficiency for Registered Nurses

This chapter will address the following platforms and proficiencies:

Platform 1: Being an accountable professional

At the point of registration, the registered nurse will be able to:

1.2 understand and apply relevant legal, regulatory and governance requirements, policies, and ethical frameworks, including any mandatory reporting duties, to all areas of practice, differentiating where appropriate between the devolved legislatures of the United Kingdom.

1.14 provide and promote non-discriminatory, person-centred and sensitive care at all times, reflecting on people's values and beliefs, diverse backgrounds, cultural characteristics, language requirements, needs and preferences, taking account of any need for adjustments.

Platform 2: Promoting health and preventing ill health

At the point of registration, the registered nurse will be able to:

2.7 understand and explain the contribution of social influences, health literacy, individual circumstances, behaviours and lifestyle choices to mental, physical and behavioural health outcomes.

Platform 3: Assessing needs and planning care

At the point of registration, the registered nurse will be able to:

3.4 understand and apply a person-centred approach to nursing care, demonstrating shared assessment, planning, decision making and goal setting when working with people, their families, communities and populations of all ages.

(Continued)

(Continued)

3.8 understand and apply the relevant laws about mental capacity for the country in which you are practising when making decisions in relation to people who do not have capacity.

3.9 recognise and assess people at risk of harm and the situations that may put them at risk, ensuring prompt action is taken to safeguard those who are vulnerable.

Platform 4: Providing and evaluating care

At the point of registration, the registered nurse will be able to:

4.4 demonstrate the knowledge and skills required to support people with commonly encountered mental health, behavioural, cognitive and learning challenges, and act as a role model for others in providing high quality nursing interventions to meet people's needs.

Platform 6: Improving safety and quality of care

At the point of registration, the registered nurse will be able to:

6.11 acknowledge the need to accept and manage uncertainty, and demonstrate an understanding of strategies that develop resilience in self and others.

Platform 7: Coordinating care

At the point of registration, the registered nurse will be able to:

7.5 understand and recognise the need to respond to the challenges of providing safe, effective and person-centred nursing care for people who have co-morbidities and complex care needs.

7.8 understand the principles and processes involved in supporting people and families with a range of care needs to maintain optimal independence and avoid unnecessary interventions and disruptions to their lives.

Chapter aims

After reading this chapter, you will be able to:

- outline the main ethical issues when working with people with mental health challenges;
- describe the ethical frameworks available to practitioners to work through complex ethical issues in practice;
- understand how ethical frameworks are applied to real-life scenarios;
- develop a critical understanding of the use of compulsion in mental health.

Introduction

Care for people who face mental health challenges involves working in partnership between the nurse and the person and family. At times, the needs that people identify may be different to those thought important to practitioners. This is when decisions need to be made about whether people can make decisions about themselves, or whether the use of legislation is necessary to provide protection for the person. These considerations are dependent on the values, knowledge and skills of people providing care, and to care well requires an understanding of the ethics and law that underpin decision making. This chapter is arranged into three sections. The first is the legal frameworks that all nurses need to be familiar with in practice. The second part of this chapter is about promoting ethical practice with an emphasis on nurses questioning the proportionality of the response to perceived risk, and the impact that force or coercion will have on the person. The third part of the chapter examines addressing inequalities in practice and provides consideration of ethical practices that promote rights through participation. The chapter aims to provide the reader with understanding of the thorny issues of consent and capacity and the underpinning principles that guide good practice. It is acknowledged that these are complex areas of practice, and therefore they need clear and systematic thinking to guide and review practice to see what met needs and provided care, and what met the needs of others, such as family members or services before the needs of service users.

This book may well be used by an international audience. In this chapter, when law is referred to, this law will be the Mental Health Act and the Mental Capacity Act used in England. The Mental Health Act in England has similar guiding principles as laws in other domains, such as the presence of immediate risk of harms and the need for a diagnosable mental illness to be present. It also holds the right to review the use of the Act and calls for consideration of the least restrictive environment, also used in mental health legislation elsewhere. In other words, the fundamental reasons why the laws are used are universal. The Mental Capacity Act is not so widespread, so the principles that underpin its use will be presented here. These include guidance about how best to include the care preferences of people who are unable to contribute directly to decisions about care. The ethical considerations are also internationally recognised, such as the principles of bioethics. Bioethics is common in nursing education and practice and has four concepts that are widely considered to provide guidance for practice. The ethics of care is included as it has a specific concern for guiding practices that address oppression, and this fits well when considering how to practise ethically when the outcome may be removing someone's human rights. The strength of the ethics of care is that it is a relational approach with an aim of collaboration through negotiation in practice so it fits well with nursing, and it can guide and review practice. The Nuffield bioethics approach to dementia is included as it is helpful to see an applied approach that is relational and collaborative to help guide practice.

The presentation of law and ethics enables a discussion of the sorts of 'rules' that guide practices when working with people who present with mental health challenges.

Equally important is how care is experienced, which is essential to understanding whether a person has had their needs met. Therefore, in the final part of this chapter we discuss the aims of ethical practice in terms of how nurses can contribute to good care for people with mental health challenges.

Mental health care and physical health care have conventionally been demarcated as different. Historically, there has been a great deal of stigma associated with using mental health services, a legacy left from the era of institutionalised care. Even now, if you ask people about assessment of a mental health problem, the response is a fear that events will spiral out of control, resulting in a loss of self-determination (Dew et al., 2007). Relinquishing control is an act of faith – that the person you are handing your fate over to can be trusted to take your preferences and needs into consideration and act in solidarity with you. For people to trust practitioners, there is a need for the demonstration of competent and skilled care – and an ability to demonstrate the values of empathy and compassion. With the introduction of the UK Nursing and Midwifery Council *Future Nurse* standards (Nursing and Midwifery Council (NMC)) (2018c), the expectation is that all nurses can respond competently and empathetically to all people who use services. Therefore, this chapter will help to develop critical thinking to meet the standards of being an accountable professional, promoting health and preventing ill health and assessing needs, planning and reviewing care. To do this, three case studies are presented and discussed throughout the chapter.

Mental health legislation

Do we need mental health laws?

Most Western countries have legislation that provides legally mandated rules for what can and cannot happen to a person with a diagnosis of a mental illness, or someone who presents as though they may have a diagnosable mental illness, and requires assessment. One key question is: why is there a need for mental health law? What would happen if mental health legislation were removed? This is in response to calls from people who use services to remove force and compulsion and improve mental health service provision. It is also beyond time we began to consider responses to people who are subjected to controls that other citizens are not (Dew et al., 2011).

Research summary

Some commentators such as Mary O'Hagan (see www.maryohagan.com/publications. php; O'Hagan, 2014), suggest that when we look back at how we treated people with mental health problems at the start of the 21st century, it is mental health legislation that we will be most concerned about, as practices will be viewed as barbaric and outdated.

Mary O'Hagan suggests that from the future, we will look back on the use of force as we do now on other outdated and unacceptable practices such as slavery, a society with a lack of care for people with certain conditions or problems, an outdated hangover from the era of asylums driven by stigma.

Activity 4.1   Reflection

Note down your thoughts on the following questions:

- Do you think that it is right that there is mental health legislation?
- What do you think would happen if there was not the option to compel people to be assessed or treated in mental health services?

As this activity is based on your own reflection, no outline answer is given at the end of this chapter.

What is mental health legislation for?

Mental health legislation has conventionally been the only law that can be used preventively to control the actions of a person to ensure they do not behave in a particular way. In essence, a mental health diagnosis can mean that controls are used that cannot be applied to other citizens within that community. So, only if a person has a mental health problem can they be detained for something they might do, rather than that they have already done. This means that fundamental rights as a citizen are dependent on health status, a situation reserved for people who have mental health problems. Is this fair? Is it right that we, as citizens, may have our rights removed based on a prediction of behaviour? Many people who have been subject to the use of compulsion such as being detained under the Mental Health Act would suggest that it is not acceptable to use force based on the grounds of risk alone. Alliances have been formed to help practitioners understand how objectionable it is to have mental health legislation used when a person is mentally unwell. Responses to this have been varied throughout the world. Other European countries have dramatically decreased the use of the Mental Health Act, such as in Italy where people are not detained under the Act but are processed through justice routes if they cause damage to property or harm another person, for example.

Primarily the criticism of mental health law is not always that it exists, but the way in which it is used. The intention or spirit of the law was to provide refuge to people at times of heightened need, but many people with mental health service challenges say that they cannot gain access to services when they are most in need, and newspapers carry stories of the waiting lists and difficulties gaining access to specialist services, such as for young people.

> ## Activity 4.2   Reflection
>
> How do you think you would respond if you found yourself being compelled to use services when you believed you did not need them?
>
> *As this activity is based on your own reflection, no outline answer is given at the end of this chapter.*

So, these philosophical questions lead us to ask: what is the purpose of mental health legislation? Legislation is used to prevent harm and to provide protection to people who are unable to maintain their own safety. However, we also know that legislation is used to help people guarantee service provision, especially when resources are tight, and an example here would be that stating a person meets the criteria under the Act secures a bed in an inpatient setting.

What is the nurse's role?

Under the new *Future Nurse* standards, it is important for all nurses to understand the legislation that affects the care of people in services, and this includes the Mental Health Act and the Mental Capacity Act. Within the Mental Health Act, there are different sections that state the activity associated with that section, such as what length of time a person may be held for, and for what purpose. It is important to remember that although the Mental Health Act is more commonly used in hospitals, it can be implemented in community settings through community treatment orders. Common sections (in England) include Section 136, which is the police holding power, that enables the police to bring a person believed to be experiencing a mental illness to a place of safety. Section 2 enables assessment of the person in a mental health facility for a period of 28 days (in England; this can be for a much shorter time in other countries, such as New Zealand). Section 3 (England) enables a person to be detained and treated for a mental illness for a period of 6 months. Part of the Act is that these conditions are explained to the person and that the person has the right to review and access to a tribunal for independent scrutiny of the implementation of the Act. In this way, the Act is intended to provide rights to the person so that they are not detained with no right to recourse. It is important to remember that people do have rights associated with legislation and nurses have a responsibility to make sure people understand their rights and how to use them.

For people who lack capacity, for example because they are unable to retain information or communicate decisions, the Mental Capacity Act in the UK provides rights of process and review. The Mental Capacity Act offers people the right to review of placement or treatment, and it provides a framework for the assessment of capacity and formal best-interests assessments for people with long-term incapacity who are unable to make decisions and a right to review of their care via inclusion in decision making. The Mental Capacity Act also ensures that practices that limit liberty are formally assessed and justified. Placing a person in a home with a locked door so that they cannot leave or providing intimate care against the wishes of the person must be planned using the Deprivation of Liberty Standards (DoLS). The principles that underpin the Mental Capacity Act are fivefold:

1. Assume a person has capacity unless proved otherwise.

2. Do not treat a person as unable to make a decision unless all practicable steps have been taken to help them – this includes accessible information.

3. A person should not be treated as incapable of making a decision because their decision seems unwise.

4. Always do things or make decisions for people without capacity in their best interests.

5. Before doing something to someone or making a decision on their behalf, consider whether the outcome could be achieved in a less restrictive way.

Activity 4.3   Reflection

What are the steps needed to establish best interests? How would you implement the five principles on a hospital ward? What accessible information do you offer people to improve their understanding of the question?

As this activity is based on your own reflection, no outline answer is given at the end of this chapter.

To ensure that nurses practise legally, it is important to remember the fundamental criteria of these laws. The Mental Health Act requires that the person has a mental illness and is at risk of harming themselves or others. The Mental Capacity Act takes the position to always treat people as though they have capacity to make a decision. It determines whether a person has capacity to make decisions for themselves, and if not, determines what the best interests of the person are and provides a process for establishing decision making. Nurses need clarity about the criteria for using the Act, and the responsibilities for informing the person, carrying out assessments and supporting people when the Act is used. It is important to remember that a person who is subject to these legal requirements can also have a say in guiding care. A person subject to the use of legislation requires more care to ensure participation in care and avoid the person becoming passive and losing control over decision making (Brannelly, 2011).

Human rights and mental health legislation

Human rights and mental health legislation have significant overlaps. It is only in particular circumstances that a state is allowed to remove the fundamental rights and freedoms of its citizens. Scrutiny is needed to make sure that mental health services are provided in a way that adheres to the law, and that people subject to them are fairly treated. The overlap between ethical concerns in practice and the Human Rights Act (UK 1998) is shown in Table 4.1.

Human Rights Act	Ethical concerns in practice
Right to life	Withdrawal of treatment
Everyone's right to life shall be protected by law	'Right to die'
	Advanced care directive
	Safe restraint practices and use of tasers
Prohibition of torture	Abuse in care, dependent upon circumstance, age and health status
No one shall be subjected to torture or to inhumane or degrading treatment	Detention under common law and mental health law
	Right to refuse treatment
Right to respect for private and family life	Removal from home without consent
Freedom of thought, conscience and religion	Right to give or withdraw consent to treatment

Table 4.1 Human rights and ethical concerns in practice

It is important to remember that legislation sets out basic rules about what can and cannot happen to a person. This is not the standard to which nursing is held to account, with much higher aspirations for how to work with people in distress, enabling participation and facilitating care where people can have their preferences for care met as fully as possible. For nurses, this raises the question of how to practise in a way that supports people in distress, to prevent harm and ensure the promotion of health.

Service user and carer experiences of compulsion under the Mental Health Act

In previous research (Brannelly, 2015, 2019), the Mental Health Act is discussed as the *boulder in the road to recovery* – using force only serves to distance the person with a mental health challenge from services, makes people not want to have contact with mental health professionals and removes trust in the relationships between people using services and service providers. Compelling a person to use mental health services continues to be highly contested on the grounds of the removal of rights, the lack of efficacy of services and treatments, creating a situation of a lack of trust of service providers, repeating trauma through coercion and a lack of informed alternatives that people who use services would welcome. Evidence suggests that people who are detained long-term in forensic settings have higher rates of suicide (Clarke et al., 2011). Major psychiatric disorders increase the risk of mortality (Craig, 2008), that is, people who have long-term and significant mental health challenges die younger than the rest of the population. Murphy et al.'s (2017) study of the experience of people detained under the Mental Health Act in Ireland identified how participants reported being disempowered and unsupported, resulting in a deleterious impact on psychological wellbeing long-term. One recommendation from that study was a reconsideration of the way that person-centred care is understood and practised in settings where compulsory detention happens and a shift to minimise the trauma that accompanies the experience of compulsion. This means that the decision to detain and compel treatment must be considered with the person's circumstances, needs and preferences, any alternatives that provide a less restrictive approach and a critical awareness of the available evidence in mind.

While there is not the opportunity to investigate in any depth the concept of risk in this chapter, it is necessary to identify it as a determinator in decisions about the use of legislation as it forms part of the criteria for the use of legislation. Risk is highly contested as a concept and holds inherent power imbalance. Assessments of risk vary between the professional and the personal. Risk assessment for predicting behaviours used by professionals has been found problematic, such as suicide assessment and predictability for completion of suicide. People who see themselves as low-risk in contention with a professional view are likely to be viewed as lacking a realistic assessment of their predicament. Glover-Thomas (2011) recognises that the 2007 amendment to the Mental Health Act in England, for example, insidiously moved to a discussion of risk that prioritised public protection over individual autonomy but that this was not intentional in practice, raising the question about the critical stance taken to legislation by decision makers in the field.

An overwhelming narrative that sits in mental health policy is the need for better access to services and service delivery at the point of need, rather than a radical rethink of how services are provided and received. This creates an impression that all is well with service delivery, but that people want more of it and easier access to it. Perhaps this narrative trope has evolved from the lack of experiential evidence regarding people who are long-term users of mental health services and who are subject to compulsion. But this raises a fundamental question about services and that is: if services are acceptable, why do people with mental health challenges not want to use them? Ridley and Hunter (2013) identified that people wanted alternatives to those they were offered and that different kinds of services would have met the service users' needs to avoid 40% of people with mental health challenges being under the Mental Health Act in England. Coercion was unwelcome and nearly half of participants thought it unnecessary. Alternatives include recovery-focused services, where peers who have their own experience are available, and there is little focus on clinical assessment and treatment (Paton et al., 2016; Johnson et al., 2018). Ridley and Hunter (2013) noted that the promises of shared power and decision making through the service user movement had not transpired into acceptable service provision, despite reviews of legislation making such claims.

A final point to make in this section is about whether some groups of service users are overrepresented in service admissions through the use of legislation and force. Barnett et al.'s (2019) systematic review and meta-analysis of international literature surmises that Black and minority ethnic groups are overrepresented in the use of legislation. This is not a homogeneous picture, with some groups more likely to be overrepresented than others. In the UK, Black Caribbean, Black African and Black (other) as well as migrants are at the highest risk of detention under mental health legislation and readmission.

Activity 4.4   Reflection

Note down your thoughts on the following questions:

* Why are some groups of people overrepresented in mental health services?
* Do you think this is social (i.e. because of poverty) or discriminatory (because the services were not set up with the group in mind) or are there other reasons why this happens?

As this activity is based on your own reflection, no outline answer is provided at the end of this chapter.

Barnett et al. (2019) commented on the typical explanations given and cautioned against unhelpful stereotypes such as increased drug use and resistance to contact with services that do not account for the disparities. Gajwani et al. (2016) conducted a study in Birmingham, UK, and warned against stereotypical explanations that are not well supported with evidence. Their conclusion was not that services are deemed discriminatory, rather that there are multifactorial aspects to the position with complex drivers at play.

Summary

Mental health legislation mandates powers to the state, enacted through mental health services, and these powers have extensive implications. People who are detained and treated without consent are disenfranchised due to the loss of control over self-determination. The concerns that people express are not unfounded and may be about medications that they do not want to take, or the consequences of being in hospital for a length of time that mean a loss of housing or contact with support networks. There are also implications that extend beyond the use of services, which people often find challenging and traumatic, and these include an inability to get insurance or being asked about detention in migration policy. The decision to use detention should only be taken when all other alternatives have been exhausted, and this in effect should make detention redundant if the right sorts of services are available and practitioners are able to creatively access the sources of help that the person needs. This raises the question of how nurses, as the professional group most frequently in contact with service users, understand the experience of mental health challenges and respond in a way that meets the nursing standards. In the next section, three case studies are included to illustrate how to approach and guide care.

Guiding principles and ethics

Nurses must work within the law, and therefore need to know the criteria for detention or treatment and advocate on behalf of service users when those are not met. Legislative requirements generally point out what cannot be done to a person, and in nursing there are higher aspirations than this to know how to work well with people, which is where ethical principles can guide practice when there are challenging situations or ethical dilemmas to work through. In mental health, the main ethical issue that is faced is the lack of consent.

Consent is a mainstay of the legal system, as it is the enactment of autonomy. Autonomy means that a person has the right to make a choice about what happens to them – to self-determine. Autonomy is enshrined in law as the guiding principle in consent. Health services are not able to provide services to a person who does not consent without good reason to do so, hence the criteria of risk of harm to self or others and a diagnosable mental illness to enact the Mental Health Act. When a person does not give consent to receive services, they are eligible to be compelled to use those services without consent as long as they meet the criteria. In practice, autonomy is not quite as clear-cut as this as a person may consent to parts of service provision but not others. For example, a person may accept being in hospital, but refuse treatment while they are there. One aspect of working with people in this situation is to encourage continuing decision making and understanding clearly what the person consents to and what they do not consent to.

Another guiding principle is whether the actions taken are proportionate to the situation. This is the principle of proportionality that is used to consider whether there was a lesser alternative that would have had less impact as a breach of human rights. An example would be that a person has intimated that they have heard voices that distress them, and they are restrained and detained for 28 days for assessment. The question under scrutiny is whether the action is justifiable given the problem. Encouraging autonomy through decision making and ensuring the response is proportionate provide two key questions about the response taken to the situation.

In bioethics, autonomy is one of the four key principles – the others are non-maleficence, beneficence and justice. As discussed above, *autonomy* is the right to self-determination through decision making about one's life. In mental health practice, this may be directly challenged because autonomy is removed about particular decisions. This does not mean all decisions, and lacking autonomy in one area does not mean that the person is globally incapable of making decisions and is often well placed to make decisions about other areas of life. In respect of autonomy, the following questions may be posed: what is the preference of the person? If this is not the course of action, why not?

Non-maleficence is the intention to practise without doing any harm. In mental health practice this means that nurses are competent in responding to the person they are caring for, skilled and working within their limitations. More broadly, it may prompt the question about whether the actions taken are harmful in any way, and whether there are alternatives that are potentially less harmful. An example here may be that it is judged more harmful for a person to remain detained in long-term care in hospital than to be discharged to care in the community.

Beneficence is the principle of doing good through care, and is what it is expected that care achieves, although this may sometimes not be the case. In practice beneficence can prompt the question of whether there is any more that can be done to benefit the person receiving care at this time. This question needs to be proportionate in that it asks this in the question of the resources that are usual in the situation. This segues into the question of *justice*, which may prompt the question about whether the care provided for the person is fair when compared to others in a similar situation, or when compared to the usual standard of care for another group. An example here is where usual provision of care is questioned for older people when compared to the allocation of resources available for younger people in similar circumstances. On an individual level, it may require examination of the response provided to others in a similar situation to ensure there is equity in provision.

Ethics of care

Brannelly (2016) has advocated the use of the ethics of care to guide and review mental health practices for marginalised groups, and has applied it to the care of people with dementia and people who are detained under mental health legislation. The ethics of care developed from the work of Carol Gilligan (1982), and Joan Tronto (1993, 2013) developed the theory further to provide an integrity of care to consider caring practices. Essential to the ethics of care is that it raises recognition of marginalisation, hence its fit with applying it to the care of people with dementia or people who are detained under mental health legislation. Raising recognition is important as it highlights the experiences that people have who are faced with these challenges, whilst also questioning whether the responses provided are adequate and proportionate. A second essential part of the ethics of care is that it values interdependence over independence and dependence. This is because when a person is dependent they are viewed as having less worth in a society that values productivity and ownership, and this is a challenge to citizenship as people may be viewed as less than human (Brannelly, 2016). The emphasis on interdependence sees all people as needing care and values care in everyday life. According to Tronto (2013), the phases of caring are:

- *Caring about: attentiveness*: at this first phase of care, someone or some group notices unmet caring needs. If attentiveness is not present then the other elements of care ethics cannot be practised. Openness, recognition, respect for identity and diversity are required. In care situations the needs of all are noted, and the course of action taken can be measured against these to understand whose needs have been met.

- *Caring for: responsibility*: once needs are identified, someone or some group has to take responsibility to make certain that these needs are met. Assuming responsibility to act on the basis of the needs identified in attentiveness requires 'judging with care', applying the ethics of care to the process to consider the direction care takes and what outcomes are likely. Attempting to meet, but not actually meeting, needs indicates a failure of responsibility.
- *Care giving: competence*: the third phase of caring requires that the actual care-giving work be done competently and with skill. Competent care requires the allocation of adequate resources, and having access to services available to meet needs at a time when they are required.
- *Care receiving: responsiveness*: Once care work is done, there will be a response from the person who has been cared for. Observing that response and making judgements about it (for example, was the care sufficient, successful, complete?) is the fourth phase of care. Note that while the care receiver may be the one who responds, it need not be so. Sometimes the care receiver cannot respond. Others in any particular care setting will also be in a position, potentially, to assess the effectiveness of the caring act(s). And, in having met previous caring needs, new needs will undoubtedly arise.
- *Caring with: solidarity*: this final phase of care requires that caring needs and the ways in which they are met are consistent with democratic commitments to justice, equality and freedom for all. Trusting and empathetic relationships are required.

More recent ethical frameworks represent a mixture of bioethics and ethics of care principles, such as the Nuffield Council on Bioethics' (2009) *Dementia: Ethical Issues*. The following components of care incorporate ethical practice that aims to be relational (as in the ethics of care) and promote autonomy and fairness (bioethics).

- *Component 1: a care-based approach to ethical decisions*. Ethical decisions can be approached in a three-stage process: identifying the relevant facts; interpreting and applying appropriate ethical values to those facts; and comparing the situation with other similar situations to find ethically relevant similarities or differences.
- *Component 2: a belief about the nature of dementia*. Dementia arises as a result of a brain disorder, and is harmful to the individual.
- *Component 3: a belief about the quality of life with dementia*. With good care and support, people with dementia can expect to have a good quality of life throughout the course of their illness.
- *Component 4: the importance of promoting the interests of both the person with dementia and those who care for them*. People with dementia have interests, in both their autonomy and their wellbeing. Promoting autonomy involves enabling and fostering relationships that are important to the person and supporting them in maintaining their sense of self and expressing their values. Autonomy is not simply to be equated with the ability to make rational decisions. A person's wellbeing includes both their moment-to-moment experiences of contentment or pleasure and more objective factors such as their level of cognitive functioning. The separate interests of carers must be recognised and promoted.

- *Component 5: the requirement to act in accordance with solidarity.* This is the need to recognise the citizenship of people with dementia, and to acknowledge our mutual interdependence and responsibility to support people with dementia, both within families and in society as a whole.
- *Component 6: recognising personhood, identity and value.* The person with dementia remains the same, equally valued, person throughout the course of their illness, regardless of the extent of the changes in their cognitive and other functions.

To be an accountable professional all actions must be justifiable, including the decision to take no further action. Ethical frameworks and principles offer a way to guide and review decision making in practice. Using ethical principles enables a consistent and systematic approach to making decisions and communicating them to other practitioners in a multidisciplinary setting. In the next section, we will bring these principles alive by applying them to the case studies.

Lawful and justifiable good practice – applying ethics to case studies

As has been stated previously, nurses must work within the law, so it is necessary to know the criteria for the Mental Health Act and the principles of the Mental Capacity Act and the rights that are enshrined in the Human Rights Act or local equivalents. This is necessary so that the rights that are compromised are only done so to provide protection and the promotion of health for the individual, and that the actions taken by services are proportionate to need. So far, so clear. However, the challenges and moral questions associated with the implementation of rights-compromising practice come from whether all of the available actions and interventions have been offered and how mental health services have worked in a recovery orientation and with a least restrictive intention. As we saw earlier in the chapter, service users whose rights are less compromised have better outcomes in services. So, the question is: how do we make sure that we are achieving this in practice?

Ethical frameworks provide the answer to this question as they enable a systematic consideration of practices. In the case of the ethics of care, it can guide as well as review practices. Bioethics is helpful for having a team discussion as they are the ethical principles most known to the different disciplinary actors involved in decisions about care. There is also another imperative that we suggest nurses consider in practice, and that is when faced with a situation in which the person does not consent to engagement or treatment, that *no stone is left unturned* (McAuliffe and Chenoweth, 2008). McAuliffe and Chenoweth (2008) set out a number of concerns that should be critically considered at each stage of decision making, in particular calling for a consultative approach and one that is culturally sensitive. This means that all of the people who can be consulted are asked about what may happen and what a good outcome may look like for the situation. Cultural sensitivity can include the very localised conditions of preference for the people involved – what is usual for them – rather than a judgement against other norms that are inconsequential in that situation. To complete this chapter, these principles will be applied to the case studies.

The first point to make is that the case studies happened in practice and are 'real' with changes to names or other defining characteristics to maintain anonymity. The authors had contact with the people involved as practitioners or as researchers. We advocate that further considerations were made before the restrictive practices that occurred were realised, because it was thought that the detention pathway was taken with stones left unturned. The key points for critical reflection are whether all available options were explored, whether services made sufficient effort at engagement and whether the assessments were valid to justify the outcomes.

Case study: James

James (32) is known to the local mental health team and has had repeated episodes of psychosis since he was 17. This means he tends to have some fixed delusional ideas about who he is and his role in the world, including that he has healing powers. He normally takes anti-psychotic medication in the form of a monthly depot injection, which he does not like but tolerates, but he has not had this for the past 2 months and has not responded to the team's attempts to speak with him. The team has contacted him by phone and called at his address on one occasion and left him a note there.

Police are alerted by a member of the public to James being in a distressed state in the centre of town, shouting and taking off his clothes. Police officers use Section 136 to take James to a hospital, where a Mental Health Act assessment is completed. James' family are no longer in contact with him on a regular basis but do attend when called by the psychiatrist to support James during the assessment. They agree that James should be detained. James tells the assessing team that he is the Messiah and has been sent to spread the word of God. This has been a common belief for James when in a psychotic episode. The mental health team who know James see that he has lost weight, probably about 10 kg. James has not been taking his medication for his high blood pressure, which currently reads at 145/80 mmHg. James says he does not need to take any medication as God has given him immunity to all human diseases. He says that his purpose is to die and be resurrected, like Jesus.

The assessing team consider that James is at risk of self-neglect as he is unwilling to take medication and that his safety is at risk due to the behaviours in the town centre and that James is unable to see this as problematic at present. They are concerned for James' mental and physical health, as well as his safety, and he is detained under Section 3 of the Mental Health Act to remain in hospital to reinstate anti-psychotic medication. He does not consent to take medication and the decision is made to enforce this under the Act. James is restrained to be given the first depot injection that day.

Activity 4.5 Critical thinking

Once James has been given the medication, he begins to say less about being the Messiah and being immune to human disease. He is referred to a cardiac clinic, where you meet him and assess his current electrocardiogram and blood pressure. How can you assess James' thinking about his situation and what part does this play in his ability to self-manage?

As this activity is based on your own critical thinking, no outline answer is provided at the end of the chapter.

Caring for James

In James' situation, the key point of care is that he had no advocate to support him in his situation. Both the assessors and James' family agreed with detention and reinstatement of medication. An independent advocate might have provided a challenge to the implementation of the Act and the reinstatement of the medication. Where family have little contact with the person it should be considered that they may not be the person of choice for support and an alternative could be identified, for example through an advanced directive. This may well be a person who James has recent and daily contact with and may not necessarily be a member of his family.

Other aspects of the care that could be contested include the risk to physical health. James is refusing to take medication for his blood pressure, but he has also lost weight. It is not clear whether the weight loss is intentional, an attempt to control his blood pressure or another aspect of the side effects of medication – for example, weight gain and metabolic syndrome are associated with anti-psychotic medication. It may be that James wants to step away from taking the medication through a depot injection to oral medication that he has more control over. Many people feel drowsy taking anti-psychotics, and that is often the main reason why people want more control over them, or take a view to stopping the medication at some point. This is a reasonable position to take. Assessment for James would include history taking, a physical assessment and review and any relevant tests.

Finally, for James, if care is to be culturally sensitive then it is prudent to examine the beliefs that he discusses, which are religious in orientation. Exploring James' understanding of these ideas is necessary to understand more about what they mean to James. Transformations, for example, are often connected to wanting a different kind of life; being a messenger from God might be connected to a feeling of worth or status. So, it is important to know what this means for James, to explore behind the statement to find the meaning for the person. Often, this is best undertaken with the support of someone who has experienced something similar and come through to work out what it meant. Overall, the approach is to prevent detention and work with James to understand more about what he wants to achieve and how he may be supported to do so.

Understanding the situation from James' perspective is likely to help in engagement with him, and therefore with a meaningful assessment that leads a nurse to know more about how to present self-management strategies that may help James see immediate and long-term improvements, thereby building trust. In non-mental health settings, being able to engage the person in this discussion informs how to approach and work with the person to achieve health and wellbeing.

Case study: Ashley

Ashley (41) has been seeing a community mental health team since she experienced postnatal depression after the birth of her second daughter 2 years ago. Six months after her daughter was born, she had thoughts of harming herself and both children, which she found very distressing. She went to her general practitioner (GP) at the time to get help. For the past 18 months she has attended appointments and responded well to a medication, fluoxetine. She has been well supported by her partner, Shania, and an extended network of friends and family. She has linked her response to past trauma as a child and has received therapy, which was challenging but helped. She now sees her mental health team every 6 weeks. Three weeks ago, she missed her appointment with her nurse, Calvin. Calvin has not been able to contact Ashley and is concerned, as last time they spoke she was feeling low in mood and not enjoying things as much, describing what she was going through as a rough patch.

Calvin calls to visit Ashley at home. Ashley's aunt, Jena, answers the door and invites Calvin in. Jena tells Calvin that Ashley has been in bed for the past 2 weeks; she is unable to look after the children or herself. She is completely demotivated to the point where she is unable to get to the toilet and is incontinent sometimes. She has no appetite, eats very little and only drinks water occasionally. When Calvin talks to Ashley, she says she is trying to stay alive. Jena says Ashley did not want the mental health team to know she was unwell as she fears her children will be taken into care. As Shania is currently working away, Jena has temporarily moved in and has been caring for the children. When Calvin sees Ashley in her room, she speaks to him for a few minutes but then pulls the covers over her head. She asks Calvin to leave her and her family alone. Her bed clothes are soiled, and Calvin is worried about Ashley, that she is at risk of continuing to neglect herself. As Ashley does not want to engage with mental health services, she is assessed under the Mental Health Act and detained under Section 2 as being a risk to herself and having a diagnosable mental health problem – depression.

Activity 4.6   Critical thinking

Ashley is moved to hospital. Within a few hours of being on the ward, she attempts to take her own life by cutting her wrists and is admitted to accident and emergency, where her physical health and her wounds need to be assessed. How would you approach this assessment with Ashley?

As this activity is based on your own critical thinking, no outline answer is given at the end of the chapter.

Caring for Ashley

In Ashley's situation, the engagement and support of family are key. Ashley is clearly struggling with her mental health at the time she is assessed, unable to get up, eat, get to the toilet, get dressed or complete daily tasks of living. The mental health team has not made contact for 3 weeks past the time of her last appointment, which suggests there was not a high level of concern. Her family have not approached services to call for help, but have put into place interventions through family support, in particular to make sure the children are cared for. In addition, Ashley does not state that she wants to die, as would be expected if a person is depressed (suicidal thoughts are key criteria for a diagnosis of a depressive disorder); she states that she is trying to stay alive. On further exploration, it may be that Ashley can explain how this is happening for her at the moment. Sensitively supporting Ashley to be at home while working with her to develop a treatment plan may be a more effective solution than removing her from the family home. Rather than Ashley moving to hospital on a Section 2, an outreach team may be a better option for quicker recovery at home. As it happened, though, Ashley was admitted and then attempted to take her life. There is an obvious need to find out why this occurred. In your assessment of her physical state, Ashley's consideration of her body and wellness or neglect may well be influenced by these fundamental fears that have a strong root in her past. Treading carefully to enable Ashley to consider her path to recovery would help promote her health and prevent further ill health.

Case study: Jerry and Linda

Jerry (67) and Linda (64) live on the outskirts of a city in the south of England. Jerry has had early-onset dementia for the last 4 years, which became apparent when he was still working as a security guard at the cathedral, mainly helping international tourists find their way around. Linda has had agoraphobia for many years, and Jerry always went out to do the errands, to get the groceries and shopping. Recently Linda has also been in recovery from cancer, which has understandably been a difficult time for the two of them. Jerry is aware that he has dementia and knows who his consultant is and that he is part of a research programme that aims to find out the cause of his early-onset dementia. He is part of another research project that looks at the usability and acceptability of global positioning systems (GPS) for people with dementia. Jerry is pleased to have his GPS as he loses his way around the city, even in the areas he knows well. Linda uses her laptop to track him and calls the police to retrieve him if he is heading in the wrong direction. Jerry talks about the police bringing him back home when he goes out at night or heads the wrong way on the bus, which he does not mind.

A friend of the family tells Linda that Jerry is not safe crossing a small but busy road at the end of the street where they live. Linda informs the community mental health team, who conduct an assessment and decide he does pose a risk to himself and others because he may walk out in front of traffic. (This assessment is not done with Jerry outside, but with the family friend, which raises some questions of fairness.) To provide alternative activities for Jerry, it is decided that he will attend a day centre at the local care home. It also happens to be where his mother is placed as she has dementia too and this is a difficult placement for Jerry to accept. He does not want to go as he does not see himself as progressed in his dementia. Jerry states he is not a risk going out and will be more careful when using the roads. He is then assessed as lacking capacity to make that decision. This prompts a best-interests conference under the Mental Capacity Act and it is deemed that it is the best course of action for Jerry, so he is taken to the centre 5 days a week. Both Jerry and Linda see that this makes Jerry low in mood and refer to it as a necessary evil in their lives. Jerry continues to ask for other activities away from the day centre. A conversation starts about whether Jerry should move to the care home full-time to avoid the distressing scenes every day when he does not want to board the bus and pleads not to go to the day centre.

Activity 4.7   Critical thinking

Jerry attends general practice every 6 weeks, where he sees a nurse who assesses his physical health. She notes he is losing weight and has low blood pressure. How would you approach this assessment with Jerry?

As this activity is based on your own critical thinking, no outline answer is given at the end of the chapter.

Caring for Jerry and Linda

Central to the situation for Jerry and Linda is Jerry not wanting to attend the day centre or move into permanent care. The implementation of the day centre was in response to the concern that was raised that Jerry might not be road-safe, and therefore should not be going out. There are two issues here. The first is that there was not a sufficient assessment of Jerry's road safety as this would require going out with Jerry to find out whether he was able to negotiate traffic and roads safely. Unfortunately, many assessments about being outdoors for people with dementia are still not taken outdoors, and this means that the assessments on which changes in care are based lack validity. The second issue is that if a person was to be found not to be road-safe, what should the response to that be? Perhaps the response needs to be that Jerry is supported to go out safely in the community by employing a support person to help him. Jerry's purpose was to do the shopping and other errands, which helped him be useful and be able to continue his purpose of supporting Linda.

If Jerry was unsafe and unable to be supported, then offering a number of service responses and seeing which were acceptable to Jerry would be the next-level response required. Helping Jerry to understand why he might need to use the service, what benefits this would hold for him and Linda and exploring the acceptability of services with him would show some sensitivity to his position.

The key points here are whether the assessment would stand up to scrutiny, and whether all available alternatives had been explored. Jerry requires an advocate to be heard, and it may well be in an alternative setting such as a GP practice that this advocacy may be found. In addition, there are physical consequences to Jerry's health as a result of the decisions that are made that affect Jerry's life fundamentally on a day-to-day basis. The components of the Nuffield approach, such as the belief about the quality of life with dementia, would be a good justification for challenging some of the implications of the decisions affecting Jerry's life, and would act in solidarity and recognise Jerry's personhood. The role for nurses is to consider the accuracy of the assessment that is undertaken, and when working with people who find it a challenge to communicate, ensuring that people trusted by the person are also able to contribute.

These case studies are illustrations of good care from a team of health professionals. The care is guided by the ethics of care and a concern for people to be able to practise autonomy. Nurses understanding these bigger-picture concerns are able to formulate approaches that are person-centred and rights-based. Good practice that provides support needs to be thought through on an individual basis for what is best for that person and the people who support them. Use of legislation should be prevented as far as possible, and only used as a last resort for the protection of the person and of other people if a risk is identified.

Chapter summary

Nurses need to know the legalities of practice to ensure competent and safe practice. Ethical principles and frameworks provide tools to think through and consider how to approach situations to promote care and health. There is a need for all nurses to understand the experience of the person and to understand more about how to help and support people with mental health challenges. This means knowing if a person's needs have been met. Central to this is the ability to support interventions with an individual's family and support network – they will be continuing to care long after the mental health team has withdrawn. All nurses must understand that every time legislation is used, it is potentially prolonging contact with mental health services and leading to poorer outcomes, and they should adopt a critical perspective to the need for force and compulsion.

Further reading

Wintrup, J, Biggs, H, Brannelly, T, Fenwisk, A, Ingham, R and Woods, D (2019) *Ethics From the Ground Up: Emerging Debates, Changing Practices and New Voices in Healthcare.* London: Red Globe Press.

This book is intended for nurses working in various fields to consider the ethics of working with people in particular circumstances and provides real-world examples of ethical questions in practice. It is a partnership between people with experience, academics and practitioners. Expanding on the traditional approach, the editors bring together a range of new perspectives on ethics that reflect the real-life experiences and interests of those who work in health and care.

Chapter 5 Supporting people with mental health concerns

Steve Trenoweth and Sue Baron

4.4 demonstrate the knowledge and skills required to support people with commonly encountered mental health, behavioural, cognitive and learning challenges, and act as a role model for others in providing high quality nursing interventions to meet people's needs.

4.8 demonstrate the knowledge and skills required to identify and initiate appropriate interventions to support people with commonly encountered symptoms including anxiety, confusion, discomfort and pain.

Chapter aims

After reading this chapter, you will be able to:

- explore various strategies that could be employed by the adult nurse to help deliver person-centred care to people experiencing mental health challenges;
- understand how mental health challenges affect communication;
- understand how to communicate with people supportively and effectively.

Introduction

Communication is a core skill of nurses and regardless of the setting within which we work, we must be mindful of unintended communication (which may undermine the messages we wish to send) and mindful of how we can use our skills to communicate effectively with our patients (which may promote the messages). We must also be receptive to the communication which our patients, clients and service users are sending to us, and sensitive to how their symptoms and wider health care experiences might undermine the messages they intend to send. This chapter will explore various strategies that could be employed by the adult nurse to help deliver person-centred care to people experiencing mental health challenges.

The focus will be on the skills of communicating and relating to people. It will build on previous chapters which explored the person-centred *recovery approach* and how this can be used as a framework to underpin all nursing interventions, stressing the importance of partnership working and using a strengths-based approach. The therapeutic approaches we will cover range from general supportive care through to more structured psychosocial interventions, and in particular we highlight a number of mental health therapeutic interventions mentioned in the new nursing curricula:

- motivational interviewing (MI) techniques;
- solution-focused therapies;
- de-escalation techniques;

- cognitive behavioural therapy (CBT);
- distraction and diversion strategies;
- reminiscence therapies.

How mental health issues affect communication

As we saw in Chapters 1 and 3, the relationship that mental health practitioners attempt to develop with service users is person-centred, based on partnership and collaboration. This is important as it affects not only the way in which mental health care should be offered but the very way in which people experiencing mental health challenges should be supported. However, at times such communication may be challenging due to the experiences of the service users and the challenges they may be facing. This is not to say that all people who experience mental distress may not necessarily have a formal psychiatric diagnosis. Not everyone who is mentally distressed has a diagnosable mental health problem and, of course, vice versa. As nurses, we should not be guided by whether or not a person has received such a diagnosis and rather should be more concerned with the person's immediately presenting needs.

Activity 5.1   Communication

Consider a patient or client you have worked with who seems to be low in mood. What made you think that they were experiencing a low mood? How did you try to communicate with this person? What were the challenges for you?

In addition to the information below, an outline answer is given at the end of the chapter.

First of all, let's consider how we communicate with a person who is low in mood. It might be that the person has a formal diagnosis of a *depressive episode*. Here, an understanding of this diagnosis may be helpful for the nurse to appreciate the patient's internal world. This will then, in turn, affect how we may be able to offer support.

It is important for the nurse to understand the difference between feeling 'down' and being depressed. For example, the *International Classification of Diseases for Mortality and Morbidity Statistics,* 11th revision (ICD-11) (World Health Organization (WHO), 2019) describes different forms of depressive episodes of varying severity – from 'mild' to 'severe' episodes (which in the latter case may be accompanied by strange beliefs and bizarre behaviour, sometimes referred to as 'psychosis').

The symptoms of a depressive episode can include:

- feelings of sadness and despair;
- a loss of sense of hope for the future;
- appetite disturbances, often with weight loss;

- sleep disturbances;
- social withdrawal;
- loss of interest or pleasure in activities that are normally pleasurable;
- decreased libido;
- decreased energy;
- an inability to concentrate;
- feelings of guilt;
- suicidal thoughts.

A diagnosis of a depressive disorder can only be made if many of the above symptoms: persist for a period of time (typically at least 2 weeks); are abnormal for the individual; present for most of the day (and almost every day); and are largely uninfluenced by environmental circumstances (WHO, 2019).

Communication with the person who is experiencing mental distress poses significant challenges for all nurses. People who experience a depressive episode, for example, typically appear very sad, but they may also be very anxious or even angry. They may not wish to communicate with others and may even actively avoid social interactions. There is always a danger that in busy health care environments, the needs of such people may be overlooked. The nurse must ensure that the person who is low in mood is not neglected and must make every effort to engage with the person. People who are low in mood also tend to have a problem with processing information, so that it may take more time than normal for the person to understand what has been said to them, and to think of a response. It is thought that this is due to either a depletion of certain chemicals (known as neurotransmitters) which facilitate the flow of information in the brain or the inability of neurons to fully utilise neurotransmitters, which again reduces the brain's ability to function effectively. This can lead to conversations with such people taking longer than usual. The problem is that there is a tendency when we are busy or pressured to try to seek quick answers, particularly in very acute settings, but with the person who is low in mood this is not usually possible. We would advise you not to rush the process, as this will not be helpful. It is most likely that the person who is low in mood will still be processing the initial question whilst you are asking the second one. So, when talking to a person who is low in mood, it is important to consider how many questions you ask and how frequently you ask them. This is known as *pacing*.

We should also be aware that sometimes when people are unwell (physically, mentally or both), their ability to comprehend what is happening to them may be diminished and they may seem less tolerant to frustration. This may include the symptoms of pain, breathlessness or confusion. There may be anticipatory fear surrounding a diagnosis or a concern about a health problem which they or a loved one may be facing. They may be frustrated by the inability of health care staff to give reassurance or answers to their questions regarding the cause of their illness or the trajectory or prognosis of a disease. In short, the person may be experiencing considerable stress or distress. The social conventions of interpersonal communication may be challenged at such times and the nurse needs to have empathy with, and an understanding of, the emotional experience of their patients. It is important to be able to recognise and anticipate that people may have such experiences, and that we consider how to communicate with people who may be on edge and therefore more prone to emotional outbursts.

How to communicate supportively

In the Nursing and Midwifery Council's (NMC's) *The Code* (2018b), emphasis is placed on prioritising people and this is demonstrated not only in the manner of our care but also in the way that individuals are communicated with and supported. The NMC requires registrants and nursing students to:

> *put the interests of people using or needing nursing or midwifery services first. You make their care and safety your main concern and make sure that their dignity is preserved, and their needs are recognised, assessed and responded to. You make sure that those receiving care are treated with respect, that their rights are upheld and that any discriminatory attitudes and behaviours towards those receiving care are challenged* (NMC, 2018b, page 6).

Furthermore, *The Code* also requires us to consider people as individuals and preserve their dignity and in so doing:

> *treat people with kindness, respect and compassion; make sure you deliver the fundamentals of care effectively; avoid making assumptions and recognise diversity and individual choice; make sure that any treatment, assistance or care for which you are responsible is delivered without undue delay; respect and uphold people's human rights* (NMC, 2018b, page 6).

Activity 5.2 Communication

List the key elements of supportive communication. How supportive do you feel your communication is with patients and clients? What do you do well in supporting people? What areas do you think you would like to develop and enhance? How might you go about this?

An outline answer is given at the end of the chapter.

The NMC (2018b) further states that we must ensure we listen to people about their wishes and their concerns by working in partnership with them, recognising and respecting the contribution that they can make to their own health and wellbeing, empowering them to become involved in decisions about their own care and recognising when people are anxious or in distress and responding compassionately and politely. Not only are these essential components of professional nursing practice, but they are also important measures by which we can demonstrate supportive communication.

There are several key principles which are important to be aware of when attempting to ensure your communication with mental health service users is supportive. These principles involve being able to manage oneself; building therapeutic relationships; communicating effectively, both verbally and non-verbally; and maintaining good professional boundaries (NMC, 2018b). We will now take a look at each of these important issues.

Managing oneself

Nursing can be a particularly stressful and at times challenging profession. When we are busy or stressed, we may 'leak' information. By this we mean that, if we are not mindful, we can unconsciously send messages (both negative and positive) to another person, and this is particularly true of our emotions, which are mostly communicated non-verbally. This can significantly affect how our communication is interpreted and even the perceptions of ourselves as caring nurses. There may well be implications if there is a perceived disparity between what we say and how we act. We may be perceived by another person as being 'deceitful' (or 'inauthentic'). This has clear implications for building a caring and therapeutic relationship with patients/service users as the person may not trust us.

It is important to ensure that we are mindful of our own communication (both verbal and non-verbal), as well as of what is being communicated by the other person. The nurse needs to ensure that, even under very trying and stressful circumstances, they remain focused on demonstrating professionalism, care and compassion, whilst maintaining the person's dignity and acting in a way that is in keeping with what is in the best interest of their patient (NMC, 2018b). This is of course by no means easy and requires considerable expertise. In fact, it is one of the many reasons why nursing is such a skilled and valuable profession – we respond not only to the physical needs of our patients, but also to their psychological and emotional needs. And we demonstrate this by our supportive communication.

Nursing can at times be a very emotionally and psychologically draining profession (Waddill-Goad and Sigma Theta Tau International, 2016) and can lead to a loss of self-esteem, reduced confidence and 'burnout'. We may be attempting to explore the concerns of our patients when we ourselves are suffering. It is vital that you are offered and receive support to help you undertake your duties, whether or not you may be experiencing personal challenges. Of course, everyone has their own mechanisms for coping, but it is vital for the psychological health of the nurse that they are able to discuss any issues that may impact on their ability to function as a nurse.

The first step in managing yourself here is to acknowledge that you need support. There is sometimes a feeling that nurses should be able to cope with anything and that any stress and distress they experience is 'part of the job'. This is simply not the case and there is always a possibility that nurses who do not receive support (both practical and emotional) at times of stress are at increased risk of burnout. If you feel your exposure to personally challenging situations has led you to feel distressed, it is important that this is brought to the attention of your manager or, if you are a student, to your practice educator and/or personal tutor. Support is readily available to help you discuss your feelings and you should not feel shame or embarrassment in accessing this if you feel it is appropriate.

Activity 5.3   Support

What support do you feel you would like in caring for patients and clients who may be experiencing mental health issues? What support is available to you?

An outline answer is given at the end of this chapter.

Building therapeutic relationships

A vital principle in forming a therapeutic relationship with a mental health service user involves clear introductions – identifying yourself, explaining your role and ensuring that you understand the person's preferred method of address. This may seem obvious, but the lack of such basic information may make the person feel invalidated. It is important to convey a clear message that you are a trustworthy person, and to instil confidence that you are able to help.

Similarly, it is important to try to establish a psychologically safe and calm environment within which a relationship can develop. Establishing trust, building relationships and developing rapport must be seen as a core role for nurses, and this is particularly important with people who may be seen as 'challenging', confused or reluctant to accept treatment.

In mental health care, the humanistic work of Carl Rogers (1951), and particularly his seminal work *Client-Centred Therapy*, continues to be very influential. Rogers helps us to appreciate the essential qualities in the development of a therapeutic relationship, which include:

- *empathy*: understanding the person from his/her own point of view, in a sensitive and accepting manner;
- *non-judgemental warmth and unconditional positive regard*: accepting and valuing the person as a human being who is entitled to respect and dignity;
- *genuineness*: this is reflected in being open and having an honest and hopeful approach, with the practitioner having a therapeutic optimism in the person's abilities and potential.

In a survey of 500 people with mental health problems, Rogers and Pilgrim (1994) identified empathy, tolerance, caring and personal respect as being qualities perceived as being particularly helpful. In another study by Nolan and Badger (2005) of people seeking help in primary care for a depressive disorder, similar qualities and behaviour were identified by the patients as helpful. These include:

- being listened to and understood;
- a hopeful attitude;
- honesty;
- practitioners being supportive, nurturing and understanding;
- knowledge in the specialty of care in relation to providing information and offering treatment;
- genuine interest and efforts to monitor progress.

These behaviours and qualities restate the core elements outlined by Rogers (1951) and set the context for developing therapeutic relationships, regardless of health care setting.

A word on the use of therapeutic touch: this can be very positive in nursing practice in building therapeutic relationships. However, it must never be used in any circumstances where the action may be misinterpreted or when a person is angry, where touch may be seen as a threatening gesture.

Communicating effectively

Before we can effectively communicate with another person, we need to hear what they are saying. Listening helps us to develop an understanding of the person's point of view. It helps us to develop empathy and ensure that we respond in a supportive, compassionate and helpful way.

Once we have listened and understood, commencing and establishing our communication is an important next step. Ensure that you adopt a respectful tone, and that the dignity of the person is not compromised. Here, it is a good idea to start by asking the permission of the person to talk (Nelson-Jones, 2016). They may not want to, or it may not be the best time for them to do so.

Nelson-Jones (2016) offers much helpful guidance to promote effective communication, recommending that you pay attention to your body language. He suggests:

- adopting a relaxed and open body posture;
- leaning slightly forward;
- using an appropriate gaze and eye contact;
- conveying appropriate facial expressions;
- trying to limit distracting gestures, such as waving your hands about;
- being sensitive to a person's culture and how this should impact your communication (such as ensuring appropriate personal space).

Nelson-Jones (2016) also suggests that time is taken to encourage the person to talk. It is a good idea to reflect back to the person how they are presenting, but this must not be done in a way which is accusatory, critical or condemnatory. Simply state, for example, that the person seems low, sad or agitated. Reassure the person that you wish to try to understand their experience and listen to their problem.

Nelson-Jones also suggest the use of 'door-openers' to encourage a conversation. Often, when you do not know a person very well, you will tend to be more formal in your approach, for example:

> *Mr Jones, I can see that you are really quite agitated at the moment. Would you like to tell me what the problem is, please? I would like to understand what it is that is troubling you. I'm here to listen. Perhaps if we had a chat, I might be able to help you?*

Of course, if you already know the person, you may already have established a rapport and relationship which you can build on in a challenging situation. For example:

> *John, is there something on your mind? You seem quite agitated today. I'd really like to talk to you to see what we can do to help. Would that be OK?*

Listen very carefully to the person's responses. This is known as *active listening* – demonstrating that you are listening to the person and hearing what they have to say. You may find that this is best conducted in a quiet, comfortable room – this maintains confidentiality and helps to reduce the overall levels of stimulation in the environment. Of course, there are often other people in the vicinity who may be receiving care and treatment, who may be able to overhear your conversation. Here, some thought is needed about a suitable venue and you must be mindful of your own personal safety. If you are going to use a quiet room, make sure that the rest of the team know where you have gone. Here, the focus should be on trying to establish what is concerning or upsetting the person.

There are some techniques of effective communication which can help the person to talk. For example, you could use *reflective statements* which reflect back what the person has said and are an important skill in active listening (Miller and Rollnick, 2013; Nelson-Jones, 2016). Reflective statements can help to check assumptions about what the patient has said, clarify meaning and also allow the client to hear 'again' what they have said. *Repeating* is simply repeating what the client has said. For example:

> Patient: *I don't know what is wrong with me. Nobody is being honest.*

> Nurse: *You don't know what is wrong with you and feel that people are not being honest.*

This, of course, can be really irritating if used often (try it with a friend)!

There are other reflective statements which could also be used, such as *rephrasing* (where a remark is reflected back to the patient in a slightly different way using synonyms, for example):

Patient: *I don't know what is wrong with me. Nobody is being honest.*

Nurse: *It upsets you that people seem to be holding back information from you.*

Another core reflective statement is that of *paraphrasing*. Here, the meaning of the client's remark is inferred and reflected back, and a good paraphrase can reflect back to the person underlying meanings and emotions (Nelson-Jones, 2016). For example:

Patient: *I don't know what is wrong with me. Nobody is being honest.*

Nurse: *You feel that you would like clarity about your condition and that people should openly discuss it with you.*

Clearly, this is quite a skill which requires practice and training, but can be very powerful in getting to what may be the heart of the problem. But a note of caution here: the less you understand about the patient and their situation, the more cautious you need to be in reflecting back the meaning within their remarks – if you do not accurately reflect what people are saying, they may feel you are not listening or do not understand.

There are of course other techniques which may be helpful in trying to understand what is troubling the patient. Questioning is a useful skill, but you should always place an emphasis on encouraging the patient to express themselves and allow them to do most of the talking. 'Open-ended' questions are very helpful in this regard as they are seen to be 'door-openers' and encourage a narrative answer. For example:

- What concerns do you have at the moment?
- What's on your mind?
- What can we do for you?
- How can we help?

Closed questions, by contrast, invite brief or yes/no answers, which tend to halt the flow of the conversation and do not encourage talk if they are overused. They should be used sparingly and only when you would like a direct answer to a specific question. Examples include:

- Do you have any concerns at the moment?
- Are you in pain?

Other techniques include using *affirming statements*, which are a way of demonstrating an empathic understanding, recognition and acknowledgement of the difficulties the patient is experiencing or has experienced. They are a means of providing direct, *genuine* support and encouragement. For example:

- Things must be very difficult for you at the moment.
- I think if I were in your position, I would also find that very difficult.
- You certainly have had a lot to cope with – more than most people perhaps.

Of course, there will be a need to close the conversation and here it is a good idea to *summarise* what has been said and to acknowledge the concerns of the patient. Summarising is the process of drawing together material that has been discussed and it shows that you have been listening actively. You should always check that your summary is an accurate representation of the patient's views. For example:

> *I'd like to pull together some of the things that you have said. Let me know if I have misinterpreted something or if I have missed something out. So, you feel that … is that a fair summary? Have I left anything out?*

Of course, there are times when the person does not want to sit down and discuss what is on their mind. This is fine but give them an invitation to approach you in their own time and on their own terms to discuss issues. Sometimes, your communication may be to explain why there has been a mistake or an error or omission in their care. Here, an apology, coupled with explanations and information, swiftly and sincerely given, can resolve many issues.

Maintaining professional boundaries

It is during times of challenge due to a patient's demands, our stress levels or the business of the clinical environment that your professionalism as nurses is most tested. From a nursing point of view, we need to consider our professionalism in handling personally challenging situations and that our respect for our patients is undiminished by their behaviour. That is, we need to ensure that we maintain good professional boundaries. It is very important to ensure one's own professional and ethical behaviour and professional boundaries when attempting to manage challenging situations, and to ensure that one works at all times within the spirit and letter of *The Code* (NMC, 2018b).

Assertion is a very important nursing skill which can be a useful technique in managing challenging situations. It is important to be able to distinguish between *assertiveness* and *aggressiveness*. Assertiveness is an interpersonal behaviour that allows us to inform others of our needs whilst ensuring that the other does not feel dismissed by our assertions (Potts and Potts, 2013). There are some important ideas here – assertiveness is an honest and positive means of expressing your own viewpoint clearly whilst listening to other people and respecting their views. When we are being assertive, we may agree to disagree. This, of course, does not rule out the possibility of negotiation and compromise.

Therapeutic approaches

So far in this chapter we have looked at a general approach to start and open up conversations with others. This can be very supportive and even therapeutic. Now we will look at specific therapeutic interventions which are designed to help support mental health challenges. Broadly, these approaches are referred to as *talking therapies* – that is, approaches which are designed, through the use of therapeutic communication, to support an individual and help them change an aspect of their thinking, feeling and/or behaving which is particularly troublesome or damaging to their mental or physical health and wellbeing. The NMC (2018c) *Future Nurse Standards of Proficiency* highlight a number of important therapeutic interventions and approaches that all nurses need to be aware of and some of these are discussed below.

Cognitive behavioural therapy (CBT)

CBT is a time-limited approach that originated in the work of Aaron Beck (see, for example, Beck, 1976) and today represents a wide range of approaches which seek to address personal problems by modifying unhelpful thoughts, feelings and behaviours. It involves close collaboration between the client and therapist and places emphasis on the personal responsibility of clients to take control of and self-manage their problems, albeit with direction from the therapist, and on the client to discover and experiment with changing troublesome aspects of their lifestyle and health. CBT can be delivered in person by a therapist either individually or as a group and there are many self-help manuals, apps and computerised forms of CBT.

The key elements of these approaches typically include:

- active collaboration in the process of therapy;
- informing clients about the principles and practice of CBT;
- helping the client see the links between the environment and their thinking, feeling and behaving, how these are interrelated and how changes in one aspect can affect others (that is, for example, how a change in one's thinking/beliefs might affect feeling and behaviour);
- the development of strategies for coping, including the development of skills through experimentation, testing and rehearsal, which occurs not only in sessions but also between sessions (through 'homework');
- self-monitoring and reviews of progress made towards the achievement of health care goals;
- helping to prevent or reduce the risk of relapse by active self-monitoring and timely implementation of skills learned through previous CBT courses and sessions (such as problem-solving techniques) to promote coping.

It is a very flexible approach and may help people to cope with symptoms across a wide range of physical and mental health challenges, including cancer, heart disease, obesity, diabetes, dermatology, chronic pain, depression, anxiety and psychosis.

Motivational interviewing techniques

MI is a client-centred and goal-directed approach which focuses on enhancing a person's motivation to change a particular aspect of their behaviour which may be troubling, or which may be affecting their recovery, health or life goals. The approach includes many humanistic principles described above by Carl Rogers (1951) (including non-judgemental listening and the development of accurate empathy), but the approach is more focused on goal-directed behaviour change than non-directive counselling.

Originating in the work of Miller and Rollnick (1991), the central principle is exploring and resolving an individual's ambivalence to change and strengthening their resolve to change. For Miller and Rollnick, this ambivalence was a key barrier to change – that is, when a person may hold a contradictory view towards something. In health care, for example, a person who is contemplating smoking cessation may give all the reasons why they should give up (e.g. costs, health reasons) and this is often balanced with all the reasons for not giving up (e.g. it relaxes me, I will put on weight, I'm not sure how I would cope).

The approach has a solid and increasing evidence base as to its efficacy and is used in a wide variety of mental health and physical health promotion activities, dietary change (Berner et al., 2021) and weight loss (Barnes et al., 2021), physical activity promotion (van der Wardt et al., 2021), medication adherence (Konstantinou et al., 2020), diabetes (Maslakpak et al., 2021), chronic pain (Borsari et al., 2021) and stroke rehabilitation (Chen et al., 2020), amongst others.

MI is typically practised in a spirit described as collaborative and autonomy supporting and is designed through asking evocative questions, to help the person articulate, illuminate and explore their ambivalence to change. The approach recognises that discord may be a factor of the change process, but rather than viewing this necessarily as a pathological function of an individual, MI sees discord or resistance as a function of the possibility that the person may not be ready to change or that change may be happening too fast for the client, and they are unable to control it. The approach recognises that the patient, client or service user is the active decision maker (autonomous) and strives to explore concerns and solutions from the patient rather than telling the patient what their issues are, why they should be concerned and what they must do about it.

MI uses a variety of strategies to help people explore and resolve their ambivalence about behaviour change – these include assessing a person's readiness to change; understanding and exploring the person's ambivalence through the use of reflective statements, open and evocative questioning; exploring options for change; and agreeing goals and plans. Typically, the health behaviour change is supported by a strategy using four key communication skills identified as critically important (Miller and Rollnick, 2002), signified by the acronym *OARS*:

1. *Open-ended* questions are more likely to get the person talking and reduce the chance of falling into the trap of offering suggestions which the person challenges or dismisses. Examples of open-ended questions include: 'what might be some of the not so good things about change for you?' or 'if you decided to change, what would be the benefits for you?'

2. *Affirmations* are statements which are designed to recognise the person's efforts to change, recognise their strengths and abilities, to help build commitment and confidence to change. An example of an affirmative statement might be: 'despite all the stress you are experiencing, it is clear that you want to change and resolve this problem'.

3. *Reflective* listening involves active and attentive listening to what the client is saying, and communicates this by reflecting back part of what the person has said (this is described above).

4. *Summarising* allows the nurse to demonstrate their interest in an individual's experiences and their understanding of what has been said. Summarising is very helpful in communicating an accurate understanding of the person's world (empathy) and in building trust and rapport.

Brief and solution-focused therapies

Brief therapies are those approaches that use short-term interventions to support an individual or to screen for a particular issue which, once detected, allows for people to refer themselves or be referred to targeted, more specialist services. Brief therapies may offer minimal interventions (such as a single session of support) or the provision of a self-help manual with little or possibly even no contact with a person. Such approaches can be used in health care screening to highlight to an individual when their behaviour or health care choices are putting them at particular risk of harm (such as the Alcohol Use Disorders Identification Test (AUDIT), which is used for a person with hazardous or harmful alcohol consumption) (WHO, 2001).

Solution-focused brief therapy (SFBT) began in the 1980s and is an approach that is widely use in health care. It is based on building solutions to problems rather than on focusing on the problems themselves. The work is future-directed, helping the person to imagine a changed future and to think of creative solutions to address and cope with particular challenges and what resources may be required to help them reach their goal. This is accompanied by a supportive communication and recognition by a therapist of the attempts that people make in resolving their issues and by encouraging and complimenting their efforts to change (Iveson, 2002). The process of change is carefully monitored by encouraging the person to evaluate their current position on the road to this imagined future, usually on a scale of 0–10, where 10 equals the achievement of all goals and 0 equals the achievement of none.

There are many advantages to the use of brief therapies, not least that this approach can be a very effective use of a busy practitioner's time. Brief therapies can be very helpful in ensuring that people are directed to services which may offer them the best and most appropriate help for a particular problem, but they may in themselves be very effective therapeutic interventions in their own right – as Miller and Rollnick (2002, page 5) state:

The fascinating point is that so much change occurs after so little counselling.

De-escalation techniques

Broadly speaking, de-escalation techniques are are used to diffuse tense, conflictual situations or where a person is showing signs of agitation, irritation, anger or aggression. The National Institute for Health and Care Excellence (NICE) (2015) suggests that de-escalation should be used at the first signs of heightened arousal or conflict. Often, de-escalation is best facilitated by knowing what has been helpful for an individual previously – assuming, of course, that this information is readily available.

NICE (2015) makes further recommendations for de-escalation:

- Recognise the early signs of agitation, irritation, anger and aggression.
- Understand the likely causes of aggression or violence, both generally and for each service user.
- Attempt to empathise with the person.
- Use techniques for distraction and calming, and ways to encourage relaxation.
- Recognise the importance of personal space.
- Respond to a service user's anger in an appropriate, measured and reasonable way and avoid provocation.
- Ensure that the person is treated with dignity and respect.

De-escalation requires the nurse to use a wide range of verbal and non-verbal communication skills. This may include proactive strategies to effectively manage known 'flashpoint' situations (e.g. being unable to accede to a request). The nurse needs to be self-aware in such situations and able to adopt effective self-management strategies to control possible 'leakage' of verbal and non-verbal expressions which may be perceived as negative, such as those of anxiety or frustration. In a volatile situation, NICE (2015) advises that one staff member should take the lead role in communicating with the agitated person and that they should assess the situation for safety and negotiate to resolve the situation in a non-confrontational, accepting and non-hostile manner. Using a quiet designated area or room may also be helpful to reduce emotional arousal or agitation and support the person to become calm. However, de-escalation is a shared strategy, and it is important that clients, patients and service users too are able to recognise and manage their own triggers. While this may not be appropriate when the person is agitated, moving forwards, helping the person to recognise and manage their anger and frustration may be an important part of the person's care.

Distraction and diversion strategies

Distraction and diversion strategies comprise a set of skills which help the person to cope in challenging situations. The person may feel overly anxious, even panicky, in situations and as a result may engage in behaviour which is ultimately unhelpful, even harmful, and may serve only to perpetuate the person's distress by creating secondary problems – such as self-harm or self-medicating by using drugs and alcohol.

Distraction techniques are an adaptive and helpful way to ease tensions or intense emotions. They are a way of focusing attention away from the stressor on to something which allows the person a temporary reprieve, to decrease the intensity of the experience and allow them to take control. It is important to realise that distraction and diversion are not a permanent escape from a stressor but a way of coping for a short period of time. The person may need further support through the use of talking therapies and other approaches to understand, resolve or manage their distressing experiences. These include CBT, mindfulness and stress management techniques.

Typical distraction and diversion strategies are likely to be bespoke to the individual (that is, what the person finds works best for them) and may include:

- counting backwards from 100;
- doing some chores, such as housework, gardening, cleaning the car, and so on;
- taking some exercise or going for a brisk walk;
- listening to music, reading a good book or watching an absorbing film;
- doing a jigsaw or some puzzles or crosswords;
- doing some arts or crafts;
- talking to someone they trust.

Reminiscence therapies

Reminiscence therapies are a range of approaches which help the person who is living with dementia to connect with others in sharing their past, pleasant and meaningful experiences and personal stories with others. This helps to promote their dignity and personal worth and feel validated. The positive feelings associated with such reminiscences are thought to boost a person's mood and reduce agitation and behaviours such as wandering.

There are many different approaches that often focus on evoking memories by stimulating the senses, which may include:

- listening to favourite music;
- smelling scents or tasting favourite foods;
- undertaking familiar actions associated with previous jobs or hobbies (e.g. arts or crafts);
- touching familiar objects, such as favourite jewellery or prized possessions;
- looking at photographs or keepsakes;
- using the internet to discover more about the person's home town or significant historical events (such as jubilees, decimalisation, etc.).

These activities are the springboard to help the person recall and to chat about their experiences. The nurse would engage the person living with dementia in conversation by asking questions such as 'do you remember when...?' Or 'what was it like for you when...?' It is important to recognise that such reminiscences may evoke bad as well as good memories, so the nurse must be able to respond sensitively.

Chapter summary

In this chapter, we have explored a number of ways in which the adult nurse can support people with mental health concerns. We have looked at how mental health issues can affect communication. We have discussed how we can ensure that our verbal and non-verbal communication and behaviour can effectively and supportively demonstrate our professionalism as nurses, including how we manage ourselves and how we maintain professional boundaries. We stressed the importance of the nurse being able to access and receive emotional support. We have also explored a number of techniques which could be used in attempting to resolve challenging situations, such as the nurse's ability to manage themselves, being able to build relationships, effective communication and maintaining professional boundaries. Finally, we explored some therapeutic approaches in mental health, namely CBT, MI, solution-focused brief therapy, de-escalation, diversion and distraction techniques and reminiscence therapy.

Activities: Brief outline answers

Activity 5.1 Communication (page 80)

Often, people who experience low mood do not directly communicate that fact. This might be because they do not realise that they are experiencing low mood or, if they do, sometimes because of the nature of their experience they may not feel entitled to support, and they may have feelings of worthlessness. We often notice that people are experiencing low mood due to their overall presentation (looking sad or downcast; uncommunicative; negative ideas; sometimes people may be angry), but please note that not all people who are low in mood cry. There may be other issues you notice such as the person not eating or drinking and ultimately appearing dehydrated or losing weight. Communication with this client group can be very challenging at times – the person may be very reluctant to talk or indeed unable to talk due to their mental state. Often, people talk very slowly and their responses to your questions may take longer than would normally be expected. Time and patience are required under such circumstances.

Activity 5.2 Communication (page 82)

It would be helpful to look again at the key skills outlined in this chapter and reflect on your communication style. Feedback from patients/clients, carers or relatives is an essential part of developing your skills – try to ask them if they felt you were supportive, and in what ways. This could be discussed with your practice assessor or supervisor and recorded in your practice portfolio. It would be helpful for you to consider what skills you would like to develop; discuss with your practice assessor and/or personal tutor what educational opportunities are available to you to meet any perceived deficit.

Activity 5.3 Support (page 84)

Support for people who are in turn offering support is essential. In mental health and therapeutic care, we often refer to this as supervision. As a student, you will have access to practice assessors and supervisors, personal tutors and academic assessors with whom you may be able to discuss any issues that you might have during the course of caring for others. Our advice is never to see this as a failing or weakness but to regard it as an essential element of professional practice.

Further reading

Nelson-Jones, R (2016) *Basic Counselling Skills: A Helper's Guide* (4th edition). London: SAGE.

This is a concise and very clear overview of essential communication and counselling skills. It is focused on supporting and helping patients, clients and service users who may be experiencing mental distress and offers practical guidance for health care professionals in differing settings.

Grant, A and Goodman, B (2019) *Communication and Interpersonal Skills in Nursing* (4th edition). London: Learning Matters.

This is an excellent book which expands on the issues raised in this chapter. It also explores in more detail the potential barriers to effective communication and interpersonal skills. Other key issues discussed are cultural and diversity issues in nursing and the environmental contexts within which such skills are being demonstrated.

Chapter 6 Responding to a mental health crisis

Sandra Walker

NMC Future Nurse: Standards of Proficiency for Registered Nurses

This chapter will address the following platforms and proficiencies:

Platform 3: Assessing needs and planning care

At the point of registration, the registered nurse will be able to:

3.16. demonstrate knowledge of when and how to refer people safely to other professionals or services for clinical intervention or support.

Platform 4: Providing and evaluating care

At the point of registration, the registered nurse will be able to:

4.4. demonstrate the knowledge and skills required to support people with commonly encountered mental health, behavioural, cognitive and learning challenges, and act as a role model for others in providing high quality nursing interventions to meet people's needs.
4.10. demonstrate the knowledge and ability to respond proactively and promptly to signs of deterioration or distress in mental, physical, cognitive and behavioural health and use this knowledge to make sound clinical decisions.
4.11. demonstrate the knowledge and skills required to initiate and evaluate appropriate interventions to support people who show signs of self-harm and/or suicidal ideation.

Chapter aims

After reading this chapter, you will:

- have a more indepth understanding of mental distress and the ways it can manifest in people;
- have a more indepth understanding of why a mental health crisis can occur;

- have some more ideas of how to engage with those in mental distress;
- have more knowledge on ways we can actively support people in crisis who access acute services.

Introduction

People are whole beings. When we become physically unwell we are more vulnerable to mental distress and equally when we become mentally unwell we are more likely to have physical health complications as a result. The Nursing and Midwifery Council (NMC) standards referred to above reflect this, showing how important it is for us as nurses, regardless of field of practice, to be able to understand and interact with all aspects of a person's health. This chapter looks at defining a crisis, why this may occur and how best to support someone in crisis who presents to your care in order to contain the situation and prevent it from getting worse. We will look at communication tools to aid this and hear from patient research which outlines the qualities we can best nurture in order to ensure that we are developing into the sort of caring professionals that can provide this quality of care. We will also look briefly at risk assessment and how to support the person if they are at risk of suicide or self-harm. Let us first think about Gerard as an example of how life can become overwhelming at times.

Case study: Gerard

Gerard became diabetic in his teens, and had often found this difficult to manage; he has been admitted to hospital several times over the last 20 years in order to stabilise it. Last month Gerard's marriage of 12 years ended and his ex-wife moved to a different city with his two small children. Although he continued to work, Gerard had noticed that his self-care had reduced, his alcohol consumption was rising and his diabetes, which had been stable for the previous 2 years, was again beginning to fluctuate. Two days ago, Gerard was informed he was going to be made redundant following the pandemic due to changes in the company he worked for. The combination of these factors, exacerbated by the vulnerability caused by his lack of self-care and increased alcohol consumption, pushed Gerard into overwhelm and he took an overdose of insulin, intending to end his life. He was found by his sister, whom he had texted to wish good luck for the future, and was conveyed to hospital.

Crisis

Many definitions of crisis exist. For the purposes of this chapter, crisis is defined as the point at which mental distress becomes overwhelming or unmanageable to the extent that the experience of it disrupts everyday life, as experienced by Gerard above. It is a multifaceted process which can be understood more broadly as progressive with a trajectory, recognisable in individuals, although not always linear in progression. Crisis can represent a very negative event in life; however it can also be an opportunity for growth. People decide what would constitute a crisis for them and react accordingly based on their past experiences, levels of resilience, levels of support, and so on. Individual definitions of crisis are often not explored in mental health services, and if we are not careful we judge others' actions and reactions in crisis by our own definition of what we consider to be situations worthy of the title.

Crisis theory (Caplan, 1989) suggests that people exist in emotional homeostasis until external hazards precipitate crisis, thereafter finding that their usual coping mechanisms fail, leaving them overwhelmed. Ball et al. (2005) extended this theory and proposed that there were underlying vulnerabilities inherent in those with mental health issues. These linear models propose trajectories of crisis that do not sufficiently account for the complexity of crisis experience as manifest by the participants in one study (Walker et al., 2017). Additionally, Ball et al.'s (2005) model accepts the biomedical approach to mental ill health (or mental illness), although notes it as a potential criticism from others, thus negating or minimising the inherent difficulties faced by many who experience serious mental ill health crises which may be triggered by social, economic and health inequalities. Walker et al. (2017) take a more critical realist approach to the concept of mental illness, that many diagnoses of mental illness are subjective social constructs created in order to describe the intense distress and behaviours caused by continual and sometimes extreme difficulties with living. So whilst not ignoring the fact that symptoms of mental illness can have an endogenous basis, many of the symptoms treated by mental health services may not be caused by illness but by reactions to external factors, in line with Caplan's theory. Ball et al. (2005) also assume that those with a diagnosis of mental illness are somehow different to other people, a position that could be argued to be an example of institutional prejudice. The experience of mental health issues does not make a person fundamentally different from other people. Another criticism of both these models is the underlying assumption that emotional equilibrium is the intended goal; this may not always be the case. Bennaman (2012) adds emergency to the linear models, which is helpful in extending practitioner thinking around responding to crisis and indicates a further layer of complexity to the previous models. Ball et al. (2005) describe crisis in terms of emotions, suggesting that it is symptom worsening in mental illness that causes crisis. This assertion does not recognise the possibility that mental distress may well have been initially triggered by an external event such as abuse or bereavement and could be an ongoing reaction to trauma. Both theories miss the potential for internal triggers based on negative thought patterns which often exist in the absence of a mental illness diagnosis and, of course, there is a clear possibility that the trigger for a crisis could arise from physical health difficulties.

Four prototypical and empirically derived outcome trajectories are suggested by Bonanno and Mancini (2008) as a response to trauma: chronic dysfunction, recovery, resilience and delayed reactions. Historically services focus on chronic dysfunction and delayed reactions with some more recent focus on recovery, but still overwhelmingly the thinking on the topic is problem-based. They go on to suggest an individual differences model, recognising that the vast majority of people experiencing trauma do not exhibit psychopathology but rather have a pragmatic coping style that isn't necessarily pretty or well adapted but gets the job done. These behaviours are then often labelled as 'personality issues' when, in most cases, they are examples of outdated coping strategies which worked well in the wounding crisis but no longer serve the person's best interests.

Concept summary: power, threat, meaning framework

The power, threat, meaning (PTM) framework is a strengths-based, trauma-led framework, suggesting that people have been operating as best they can within the confines of their cultural upbringing, their biological, social and psychological experience. This framework recognises that there is no one-size-fits-all answer to explain behaviour; that a mix of factors (biological, psychological, social and environmental) influence behaviour; and that a person's subjective experience needs to be taken seriously. It considers the operation of *power* within a person's life, that that power may pose a negative *threat* to the individual, group or community, the subsequent *meaning* that those experiencing the threat make of it and the behaviour that may emerge as a response to that threat.

Four key questions are asked:

1. What has happened to you?
2. How did it affect you?
3. What sense did you make of it?
4. What did you have to do to survive?

In this way people can be seen to be actively engaging threat responses for protection and survival rather than suffering biological deficits they can do little to influence. It contains within it an implicit underlying assumption that the person concerned has been doing the best they can in order to survive the circumstances in which they find/have found themselves. In mental health care, where the predominating view of those experiencing 'mental illness' is one of incompetence and unpredictability (Sayce, 2016), this represents a fundamental cultural shift.

(Johnstone and Boyle, 2018)

Dealing with people in mental health crisis is often easier if we view them from the perspective of the PTM framework. The medical model, as discussed in Chapter 3, puts the person in a position of weakness and as a result they are not so easily seen as someone who has agency and ability. If we see in terms of strengths and abilities those in mental distress who are victims of circumstance, e.g. physical ill health, bereavement, job loss, etc., then it is less effort to begin to see a way of helping them to find a way out of their difficulties.

Case study: Jaz

Jaz came to the Emergency Department following a planned overdose of 16 zopiclone tablets taken with 12 double vodkas. She intended to die and was devastated when she woke up. She felt really ill on waking and called an ambulance because she was worried that she might have damaged herself and have to live with a disability in addition to her autism. She remained actively suicidal on waking and states that she intends to complete the job on discharge. She is reacting to over 15 years of intense isolation and loneliness and the end of a particularly difficult, short relationship with a man who had been consistently bullying her. The mental health team are due to come and see her later in the day but she thinks it will be a waste of time as they won't be able to 'cure' her autism. On approach she is very prickly and a little antagonistic.

Activity 6.1   Communication

You have been allocated as one-to-one contact for Jaz as she keeps becoming distressed and it is hoped that extra support will help her feel more settled and encourage her to stay until she can be seen by the mental health team.

Using the PTM framework outlined above, how could you engage Jaz in conversation that might help alleviate her sense of crisis?

An outline answer is provided at the end of this chapter.

One of the most effective ways of alleviating isolation is by connecting to the person concerned, if they can allow it. This can be achieved simply by being respectfully curious. Most people will talk about themselves with little encouragement if asked the right sort of questions. Asking simple engagement questions about lifestyle, where someone lives and how they got to hospital lays the foundation for deeper communication. Asking about hobbies or things the person enjoys doing may help remind them that there are things in life that are worth living for and, most importantly, actively listening to the answers and being genuinely interested is one of the most validating things you can do for someone. This in itself may help that person move slightly away from the crisis and begin to see more clearly. These types of questions can be asked at the same time as carrying out interventions, for example, whilst helping someone bathe, whilst doing a dressing, and so on. Effective and meaningful communication does not necessarily have to take a lot of time.

Patient perspective

Mancini (2007) found that transformation from illness-dominated identity to an identity of agency and competence was central to recovery in mental health. The patient holds the key to their recovery. When one person encounters another a potentially creative exchange follows, and both have unique insights to offer.

The recovery model (Chapters 1 and 3) is still considered a positive advance towards increasing patient empowerment, self-determination and independence (Walker, 2006). Taking control and responsibility for one's life and thus recovering a sense of autonomy are common themes within the model (Higgins and McBennett, 2007). The recovery model is, however, weighed down by the use of pathologising, deficit-based medical and psychiatric vocabulary, which supports old paternalistic roles (Walker, 2006). So, although recovery-oriented services are more patient-centred and use words such as self-determination, independence and community integration, there continues to be a subtext, related to context, which clearly says, 'you are different to the rest of society due to your pathology and we are the experts with the knowledge to help you overcome this pathology'. As long as this is the case, no matter how many person-centred and advanced participation models are applied, the power dynamic will remain with the professional. Often very understandable reactions to circumstances get identified as symptoms, supporting diagnoses, so strengths and skills go unnoticed in the individual (Walker, 2006). When someone is diagnosed with a mental illness a reality is created in which human beings are transformed into the mental illness, thus finding themselves trapped in a circle whereby everything is interpreted to reinforce the conceptual system. In this paradigm, patients who assert themselves are labelled resistant, under the effects of transference, manipulative, and so on.

In work with people diagnosed with post-traumatic stress disorder (PTSD), Stephens et al. (2013) found a paradigm of disempowerment and deferred responsibility which contributed to considerable breakdowns in care and resulted in readmissions which might have been avoided. As an example, they cite the fact that patients complained that the system of care was difficult to navigate but rather than simplifying the process, services blamed the patients for being non-compliant. In Tyson's (2013) study they found most staff agreed that patient involvement in care planning was difficult, although they were not clear why. They found some correlation between different staff beliefs and outcomes. Thus, those staff with a biological rather than social belief of mental distress were more likely to coerce and to encourage medication and had more negative attitudes regarding patient ability.

Patient involvement is not dismissive of practitioner expertise; rather it is an acknowledgement that professionals do not have the monopoly on wisdom. So, practitioners can offer their expertise to enable patients to use it to make decisions themselves, thus upholding more meaningful patient involvement. Patient involvement in treatment and administration decisions was one of the most important aspects affecting satisfaction of hospital care in a study by Taylor et al. (2009).

One study (Walker, 2017) found ample example of the kinds of qualities one might look for in a mental health practitioner providing care in crisis. The results, according to the placement in the data, are outlined in Table 6.1. They are listed according to three broad themes which appeared to cover the topics of validating, human and professional. In light of the fact that the therapeutic relationship is key in improving patient outcomes (Shedler, 2010; Leibman and Burnette, 2013; Harper et al., 2014), it is perhaps not surprising that the majority of the qualities fell into the validation and human categories. From this data the top seven qualities that were repeated several times across the interviews are: listening, understanding, reassuring, respectful, knowledgeable, non-judgemental and identifying self on arrival. Most of these are echoed within policy whereby patients list similar qualities as being important to being a good health care professional (Care Quality Commission, 2015).

Validating	Human	Professional
Validating	Friendly	Non-judgemental
Listening	Reassuring	Efficient
Non-dismissive	Smiling	Following the rules
Understanding	Optimistic demeanour	Identifies self on arrival
Interested – 'a real human interest'	Compassionate	Knowledgeable
	Empathic	Consistent
Attentive	Human	Courteous
Caring	'A person caring for another person'	Fair
Accepting		Balanced
Good eye contact	Normalising	Polite
	Open	Professional
	Respectful	Advocate
	Helpful	
	Amenable	
	Happy	
	Nice	
	Kind	
	Supportive	

Table 6.1   Qualities hoped for in a health practitioner

Communication skills

Already mentioned above is the concept of respectful curiosity. This approach lends itself well to providing great patient-centred care. Additional skills to be nurtured are listening and validation skills. The very act of listening to a person in distress is a validating thing to do. We are showing just by doing this that we care about them and value them enough to give them some of our time. Listening, using the active listening skills you will remember from your training, is a powerful tool in itself. If you remember a time when you were worrying about something and then talked to a trusted friend about the issue, you will no doubt recall a sense of relief that you had shared a trouble and a warmth towards the person listening. This works in just the same way for patient–clinician communication.

Activity 6.2   Revision and listening skills

Think back to the times you have learnt about active listening. Make a list of the ways you remember that you can show someone you are listening.

An outline answer is provided at the end of this chapter.

Supporting a person in distress

Part of the human condition is that emotions happen, sometimes quite quickly. There is always a good reason for this happening, but it is not always noticed or known by an observer. The listening skills outlined above are the most powerful ones to use in finding out what has occurred to make someone distressed and helping someone to become calm enough to be able to talk. There are other techniques that are also useful:

- *Being with*: this simply means being a supportive presence whilst someone is venting and allowing the emotions to subside naturally. Phrases like 'I'm here with you' or 'you're safe here' might be useful here.
- *Validation*: this means showing that you can see how difficult a situation is for them even if you do not fully understand it. Validation does not mean that you agree with them or think the same; it shows that you are making efforts to understand them and work with them to help resolve things. Phrases like 'I can see how difficult this is for you' might be useful here.
- *Simple communication*: when we are highly emotionally aroused, we cannot think as clearly and intelligently as we might otherwise do. Since this is the case, when dealing with someone who is very distressed keep your verbal communication very simple and direct if you need them to do something and focus your efforts on helping them become calm to a point where they can communicate their distress to you verbally.
- *Touch*: carefully used, touch can be a very useful way of communicating care to someone. However, when someone is highly emotional, touch can very easily be misinterpreted as a threat. Therefore, until someone has calmed enough to be asked if touch would help, it is probably best to avoid this if possible.

Risk assessment

In any health care environment there will be risks inherent in the building, the people working in it and those attending for care. In order to identify the risks and hazards in the workplace that might cause harm to patients/clients, visitors and staff, we carry out risk assessments. Employers have to carry out risk assessments of their workplaces by law, but employees also have a responsibility to be on the lookout for hazards and take action to remedy them when spotted (Royal College of Nursing, 2020).

Traditional approaches to risk assessment have tended to concentrate largely on historical risk which, whilst being valid to a point as history is a good predictor of future behaviour, over-reliance on it results in people being held back by their past. This can often lead to delayed discharge in the inpatient setting, and in a financially restricted climate this is problematic. There are associated risks of admission described by the Care Services Improvement Partnership (CSIP Acute Programme and Change Agent Team, 2007), such as increased risk of aggressive behaviour, promotion of dependence and lowering of staff morale. We all have to take risks on a daily basis, and it is unrealistic of services to expect practitioners to be able to eliminate and control risk. However, increased positive risk taking requires more complex clinical skills (Felton and Stacey, 2008). In an acute hospital environment this is likely to involve referral to other services such as a liaison team or a crisis/community mental health team.

As an adult nurse in a general hospital environment, you are most likely to need risk assessment skills when deciding when/if to refer to the mental health team and if a patient wants to leave before treatment is complete.

Case study: Toni

Toni is a 24-year-old woman who has taken an overdose of 16 paracetamol tablets in response to distress regarding a relationship breakdown. It is 11 p.m. and the mental health team in the hospital do not start work until 8 a.m. the next day. Toni is not willing to wait to see them. She has had her blood test to check her paracetamol levels but the results are not back yet. When asked, Toni states that she probably won't self-harm by overdose again but she is not willing to give clear reassurance of this. Toni is not receiving care from a mental health team in the community. She is alert, able to communicate her wishes clearly and does not appear to be experiencing any obviously concerning symptoms of mental ill health.

Activity 6.3   Decision making

Do you allow Toni to leave the department without seeing the mental health team?

An outline answer is provided at the end of this chapter.

Personal support plans

One technique that is often used in acute hospitals, particularly for patients who attend frequently with similar issues of low physical or psychological risk or patients who are very complex and need a coherent consistent response from services, is creating a personal support plan alongside the patient. This is a care plan that caters for their needs when attending the service and is used by all the professionals likely to come into contact with that person during their care episode. As with all care plans, these are most likely to be effective if co-produced and can give the patient a sense of being held and cared for in a way that minimizes the risk of high expressed emotion occurring.

Chapter summary

This chapter started by defining a crisis, why this may occur and how best to support someone in crisis who presents to your care in order to contain the situation and prevent it from getting worse. We looked at some communication tools to aid this and heard from some patient research which outlined the qualities we can best nurture. We also looked briefly at risk assessment and thought about how to manage the situation if someone is at risk of suicide or self-harm.

Activities: Brief outline answers

Activity 6.1 Communication (page 100)

At a time of crisis, it is possible that Jaz is not feeling able to talk as she may be overwhelmed, particularly if the Emergency Department is noisy and she may be more sensitive to sensory stimuli due to her autism. If this is the case, indicating that you are interested and you care by letting her know that you are going to stay with her and help with anything she needs during the time you have, repeating this periodically and then remaining quiet might be the right approach. It may not be sensible to ask Jaz how she feels at this point as following self-harm it is probably safe to assume that she does not feel very good. Therefore asking this question can antagonise. Instead asking, 'Is there anything you need?' 'Are you up to chatting?' may be more useful and elicit a better response. If she does open up and talk then asking what happened to bring her to hospital could be a good way to get into what is going on for her. Whatever issue she raises in answer, if approached with the assumption suggested by the PTM questions above, can be responded to in the belief that she was doing the best she could at the time and the acceptance that this approach allows is also very validating and likely to help her to become calmer.

Activity 6.2 Revision and listening skills (page 103)

Listening skills you may have listed are:

Verbal

- Ask open-ended questions.
- Ask probing questions.
- Request clarification.
- Paraphrase.
- Be attuned to and reflect feelings.
- Summarise.

Non-verbal

- Be attentive, e.g. lean forward.
- Maintain eye contact.
- Nod occasionally.
- Smile and use facial expressions that match what is being said.
- Keep an open posture.
- Use small non-verbal sounds like 'uh huh' and 'aah'.

Activity 6.3 Decision making (page 104)

The key to this is the level of capacity that Toni appears to have. Whilst we are instructed by the Mental Capacity Act to assume capacity until proven otherwise, in this instance there are clearly risks of repeated overdose, needing recall for possible treatment and not getting the mental health support she might need; therefore, it is important that we ascertain if she has the capacity to make this decision. As a nurse we can check if she *understands* the risks of leaving without knowing the result and the possibility of recall and the dangers inherent in not having treatment following paracetamol overdose if indicated. We must check if she has *retained* this information and been able to use it to *weigh up* the risks herself and then be able to *communicate* clearly her decision to us as health care workers. If this is the case then she has the right to discharge herself even without the blood results as making unwise decisions is not in itself a sign of lack of capacity. If it is possible to negotiate with Toni for her to stay until the blood results are back in order to facilitate treatment if needed, this would be advisable and then she could be discharged with a promise that she will see her general practitioner (GP) for follow-up. It would also be advisable to make sure that the discharge summary tells the GP that she was unwilling to wait and/or receive treatment.

Further reading

Baker, C, Shaw, C and Biley, F (2013) *Our Encounters with Self-Harm.* Ross-on-Wye: PCCS.

This book is an easy read as each chapter is written by someone with direct experience of self-harm. It is a great way to gain different perspectives on the subject from people who self-harm, carers and staff and really helps us to understand this very complex and diverse topic.

Johnstone, L and Boyle, M with Cromby, J, Dillon, J, Harper, D, Kinderman, P, Longden, E, Pilgrim, D and Read, J (2018). *The Power Threat Meaning Framework: Towards the Identification of Patterns in Emotional Distress, Unusual Experiences and Troubled or Troubling Behaviour, as an Alternative to Functional Psychiatric Diagnosis.* Leicester: British Psychological Society.

The full document is enormous; however a shorter summary version is available here: www.bps.org.uk/sites/bps.org.uk/files/Policy%20-%20Files/PTM%20Main.pdf and recently published in 2021 is a book to accompany it and make the whole thing rather more digestible. This is highly recommended. It outlines the framework, which is a strong challenge to the pervading medical model in mental health care, and provides a clear grounding in the evidence underpinning the framework.

Russo, J and Sweeney, A (2016) *Searching for a Rose Garden.* Ross-on-Wye: PCCS.

This book is another edited collection of chapters from differing perspectives that explore radical alternatives to mainstream psychiatric practices. There is a wealth of ideas within this book of ways to engage creatively with people in distress.

Chapter 7 Overview of the therapeutic use of medicines in mental health

Josie Tuck

NMC Future Nurse: Standards of Proficiency for Registered Nurses

This chapter will address the following platforms and proficiencies:

Platform 1: Being an accountable professional

At the point of registration, the registered nurse will be able to:

1.9 understand the need to base all decisions regarding care and interventions on people's needs and preferences recognising and addressing any personal and external factors that may unduly influence their decisions.

Platform 3: Assessing needs and planning care

At the point of registration, the registered nurse will be able to:

3.2 demonstrate and apply knowledge of body systems and homeostasis, human anatomy and physiology, biology, genomics, pharmacology, and social and behavioural sciences when undertaking full and accurate person-centred nursing assessments and developing appropriate care plans.

3.3 demonstrate and apply knowledge of all commonly encountered mental, physical, behavioural, and cognitive health conditions, medication usage and treatments when undertaking full and accurate assessments or nursing care needs and when developing, prioritising and reviewing person-centred care plans.

Platform 4: Providing and evaluating care

At the point of registration, the registered nurse will be able to:

4.14 understand the principles of safe and effective administration and optimisation of medicines in accordance with local and national policies and demonstrate proficiency and accuracy when calculating dosages of prescribed medicine.

(Continued)

(Continued)

4.15   demonstrate knowledge of pharmacology and the ability to recognise the effects of medicines, allergies, drug sensitivities, side effects, contraindications, incompatibilities, adverse reactions, prescribing errors, and the impact of polypharmacy and over the counter medication usage.

4.16   demonstrate knowledge of how prescriptions are generated, the role of generic, unlicensed, and off-label prescribing and an understanding of the potential risks associated with these approaches to prescribing.

4.17   apply knowledge of pharmacology to the care of people demonstrating the ability to progress to a prescribing qualification following registration.

Chapter aims

After reading this chapter, you will be able to:

*   identify the broad groups of mental health medications and the most commonly used medications in each group;
*   identify common effects and side effects of the commonly used medications, and demonstrate knowledge of how to respond to them;
*   describe the therapeutic use of mental health medications and the implications for individuals who are prescribed them;
*   understand the clinical implications for nursing practice across health care services when working with individuals taking these types of medications.

Introduction

Mental ill health is a leading cause for disability in the UK and nine out of ten adults who present to health services are seen in primary care (NHS England, 2014). It is estimated that 40–60% of primary care visits are a result of psychosocial issues (Woods et al., 2015) and so all health professionals, regardless of discipline, need to know how to support individuals with the most common life experiences that impact on mental health (Chelvanayagam et al., 2020).

With the publications of the new Nursing Midwifery Council (NMC) Standards in 2018, there has been some speculation about the term 'prescribing-ready'. Despite the apparent ambiguity of this phrase, the NMC are clear that registered nurses should be adequately prepared from their pre-registrant training to be able to progress to an approved prescribing course (NMC, 2018a).

This chapter will help you to develop knowledge of psychopharmacological treatments and their application to the care and treatment of individuals with mental ill health.

The chapter is divided into two parts. Part One will consider some of the general principles and approaches to medication management using case examples. Part Two will look at some of the most used groups of medications in more detail and their implications for nursing practice.

PART ONE

In Part One we will look at the overview and general principles of medication use for the treatment of mental ill health seen in all areas of health care practice.

General principles of medicine use in mental health

The use of medication in the treatment and management of people experiencing mental ill health can be an important factor in recovery for many individuals. This is due to the potential therapeutic effects but also because of the adverse effects. In short, the use of medication can both help and hinder the person's recovery.

Use of medication should not be a first-line intervention. If an individual's symptoms can be managed with psychosocial interventions, such as self-help, talking therapies, diet and exercise, then this is always the preferred option. Symptoms of anxiety and depression can resolve without medication, particularly if they are closely linked to external stressors or factors in the person's life and often the best course of treatment is to support the individual to consider the potential external influences and give them tools to change or manage their mental health in the short and medium term. In the absence of severe distress that is compromising a person's ability to look after themselves or concerns for the safety of the person or others, medication should be a last resort.

UK Clinical Guidelines, such as those from the National Institute for Health and Care Excellence (NICE) (available online at www.nice.org.uk) and *The Maudsley Prescribing Guidelines in Psychiatry* (Taylor et al., 2021), set the parameters for the use of medication for mental ill health. These guidelines are helpful resources for understanding the use, review and cessation of medication treatments once psychological and psychosocial interventions have been implemented. There is emerging evidence on the benefits of social prescribing (Dayson and Bashir 2014), which focuses on connecting people with a variety of community groups and services to improve their health and wellbeing. This has led to it becoming a routine part of supporting people with their mental health and its importance should not be underestimated as either a standalone intervention or alongside the use of medication. The following case study of Brendan is an example of someone who is unlikely to require medication as part of his treatment plan and who could benefit from psychosocial interventions.

Case study: Brendan

Brendan (35) has arranged to see the nurse practitioner at his general practice surgery as he has not been feeling himself for the last few months. He feels very worried about everything and on edge all the time, particularly when he wakes up in the morning. He usually enjoys his food but has not been eating as much for the past couple of weeks. He is working full-time but has been spending less time with his friends. He usually goes for long cycle rides at the weekends with friends but has been doing this less over the past month. Brendan has never felt this way before but recalls his mother always used to say he was 'an anxious child' and like his grandfather, who suffered with his 'nerves'. After a holistic assessment, the nurse discovers that Brendan has been drinking 4–5 pints of ale every evening for the past 6 months.

The nurse recommends that he reduces the amount of alcohol he drinks and gives him information on how to do so gradually. She also encourages him to go out cycling with friends again and helps him set a small goal of going twice in the next month. She arranges to see him in a month's time to see how things are going and tells him what to do in the event that he starts to feel much worse. Brendan thinks this is a good plan and is grateful to the nurse for taking his worries seriously.

In this case study we can see that the nurse has considered the impact Brendan's alcohol intake may be having on his mood and has educated him on why and how to reduce this safely. She has also taken the opportunity to reconnect him with a social hobby, which has the benefit of increasing his time exercising outdoors. These simple interventions are likely to be beneficial in lifting Brendan's mood and improving his overall wellbeing and therefore medication is not required.

There is evidence that the use of psychotropic medication, that is, medication used for mental health, is increasing (NHS Business Service Authority, 2020). The number of prescriptions for anti-depressants alone is thought to have doubled in the past decade (Heald et al., 2020), with around 930,000 people in England being continuously prescribed an anti-depressant between April 2015 and March 2018 (Public Health England, 2020). It is therefore likely that nurses working across health settings will meet people taking these types of medications.

While medication use is increasing, their efficacy remains variable and unpredictable for individuals. People experiencing symptoms of a depressive disorder, anxiety or psychosis have been well researched and therefore clearer treatment paths and prescribing guidance are available. Conversely, research on the potential impact of medication for individuals experiencing a personality disorder or post-traumatic stress disorder is still evolving. This often leads to symptoms-based treatment where clinicians will use different medication to target the most distressing symptoms the individual is experiencing. It is therefore not uncommon to find individuals on a variety of medications used in mood disorders, psychosis and anxiety despite an absence of these diagnoses. This means that, as nurses, it is important to understand not only the medication that is prescribed, but also the reason it has been prescribed for the individual under our care. Speaking to individuals about their medication can not only tell us why they are prescribed it, but also their experiences of it. What is helpful about it? What is not helpful? Do the medications have side effects? Are they easy to live with? Having these conversations leads to the person being included in the decision-making process. Shared decision making in the use of medication is a key aspect of safe prescribing (Royal Pharmaceutical Society, 2016) in all areas of health care, so involving individuals in discussions about medication options and their experiences are key to enabling informed decisions.

Legal and ethical considerations of medicines use

The use of legal processes within contemporary mental health care remains common. The consideration of these legal implications in the context of medication is therefore important.

The Mental Health Act (1983, updated 2007) is used to assess and treat individuals with a suspected or confirmed mental illness, if there are significant risks of harm to the individual or others, and in the absence of the person's consent. The Mental Capacity Act (2005) is used to assess and determine an individual's ability to make decisions regarding aspects of their health care and is indicated where individuals are not able to consent due to diminished capacity because of impaired understanding, retention and communication of their wishes. Once diminished capacity is established, decisions can be made, within the legal framework and guidance, in the person's best interest. Both key pieces of legislation have Code of Practice documents that are useful guides in all areas of health care practice where their use is common.

The implications for medication use of these two pieces of legislation are both legal and ethical. That is, what can legally be done, and what ethical considerations need to be considered alongside it. For example, the use of the Mental Health Act to detain and enforce treatment for mental health can be applied when the individual is an inpatient in a hospital setting (this excludes outpatient and emergency departments). However, just because an individual in this scenario *can* be legally forcibly given medication during an episode of illness does not necessarily mean it is the right thing to do. This can create tensions around decision making, particularly when balancing the safety of individuals or others against their wants and wishes. This is demonstrated in the following case study of Robyn.

Case study: Robyn

Robyn (57) is known to mental health services and has a diagnosis of schizophrenia, a type of relapsing psychosis. She normally takes olanzapine 20 mg daily, an anti-psychotic medication which is prescribed because she hears voices that tell her others are intent on harming her and this causes her distress. When taking olanzapine, these voices become less intense, and Robyn can employ other techniques to feel less distressed by them. Unfortunately, the olanzapine has been responsible for a significant increase in Robyn's weight, and she is concerned she is putting herself at risk of heart disease and diabetes. Robyn therefore stopped taking it to lose weight and improve her overall health. She is now saying she is no longer willing to take olanzapine due to fears it will make her put on weight.

Robyn has been brought to hospital by police officers who have used their holding powers under Section 136 of the Mental Health Act to bring her to a hospital-based place of safety for further assessment as there were concerns about her mental health. Police officers detained Robyn in the street as she was holding a knife and making threats to harm anyone who came near her, referring to alien life forms.

In this example, balancing the risk posed to others, the level of Robyn's distress and the implications of side effects is difficult. However, through discussion and acknowledgement of her fears about side effects, considering an alternative that is much less likely to cause the unwanted effects she has described would be both reasonable and ethical practice. By having this discussion and responding to Robyn's concerns, forcible treatment under the Act may be avoided. This would lead to better outcomes for Robyn and an improved experience of health services.

The use of covert administration of medication is mostly seen where a lack of capacity is established. Often this is where a cognitive impairment is present in dementia or where neurogenerative disorders such as Huntington's or Parkinson's disease occur. Decisions to use covert administration of medication are not taken lightly and are usually subject to clear processes and procedures by all involved, including family members, carers and professionals.

Activity 7.1   Reflection

Enhance your learning from these case studies, and take a moment to reflect on Brendan and Robyn's situation. Consider the following:

- If you met either person in your area of practice, how would you ensure you respond to their mental health needs alongside their physical health?
- How might your approach differ in a hospital setting versus an outpatient department or general practice?

A brief outline answer is given at the end of this chapter.

Long-term conditions and co-morbidities

In contemporary health care, it is widely agreed that the physical health and mental health of an individual must be considered together to optimise recovery (Department of Health, 2011; NHS England, 2014; Naylor et al., 2016). People experiencing long-term physical illness, particularly cardiovascular disease, diabetes and chronic obstructive pulmonary disease (COPD), are two to three times more likely to develop mental health problems than the rest of the population (Dury, 2015). Similarly, those diagnosed with mental ill health have poorer health outcomes and shorter lifespans (Majed et al., 2012; Davies, 2015; Gaglioti et al., 2017).

Despite knowledge of the prevalence of mental ill health, and its association with poorer outcomes when combined with physical conditions, a disparity remains between mental and physical health care whereby mental health issues are not regarded with the same level of importance as physical health conditions (Department of Health, 2011; Health and Social Care Act 2012; Royal College of Psychiatrists, 2013). Long-term physical health conditions have the potential to be well managed but, when combined with mental ill health, the complexity increases and arguably changes the approach needed to support people in managing their own health needs.

The National Health Service (NHS) *Long Term Plan* pledged further investment and '*a focus on long term conditions*' (NHS England, 2019, p68), including mental ill health. Improved recognition of this population group is imperative to enable health promotion, offer treatment and improve overall quality of life.

The use of polypharmacy, that is, the use of multiple medications in one individual, is a further complication for these individuals and means that as nurses we have a part to play in the careful consideration of how to use medication. Having an overview of the clinical picture of someone's physical and mental health is essential because of the increased potential for interactions between medications, medication and disease processes and medications and food or substances such as alcohol and nicotine.

The case study of Amir gives an example of how nurses can play an important role in supporting people with both physical and mental health long-term conditions.

Case study: Amir

Amir (25) sees his practice nurse for his annual asthma review. He appears breathless and anxious throughout the appointment. Amir tells the nurse that he has social anxiety, which has become worse since he started a new job. His asthma has also become worse even though he continues to use his inhalers as directed. He is experiencing panic attacks, particularly in the morning shortly after he leaves for work.

(Continued)

(Continued)

The nurse takes a thorough history and asks Amir whether he has been using any other medication apart from his inhalers. Amir shares with the nurse that he has been using some of his mother's propranolol, which she is prescribed for anxiety, to help him in the mornings because he doesn't want to lose his job. The nurse checks the *British National Formulary* (BNF) and discovers that propranolol can exacerbate asthma. She shares this with Amir, and he agrees to stop taking the medication. They plan for how else he can try to manage his anxiety and agree to meet in 1 week to review how things are with his physical and mental health.

When he returns, Amir is no longer using propranolol and his breathing has improved. His anxiety is still problematic and so the nurse suggests he refer himself to his local NHS service for first-line treatment in the form of cognitive behavioural therapy (CBT).

In the case of Amir, the nurse has recognised that both his anxiety and asthma are at play here and has responded by conducting a thorough assessment to understand what is happening for him. Incidents of people using the medication of close friends or family members are not uncommon throughout the population and it is therefore important when asking about medication to ask about anything the person might be taking, regardless of whether it is prescribed, procured over the counter or obtained through other means. Here, the nurse has been able to correctly identify a medication–disease interaction through gathering information in an assessment and checking reliable information on the use of propranolol. She educates Amir about this and agrees a plan with him to improve the symptoms of his asthma. Alongside this, she acknowledges his social anxiety and considers what may be helpful to him, caring for Amir holistically.

Management of adverse side effects

Side effects, that is, adverse effects from medication, are common and can significantly impact on the recovery of an individual. As such, being able to identify and respond appropriately to these unwanted effects is an important role for the nurse, who is likely to either observe them or have the side effects reported to them as someone working closely with service users.

The experience of side effects of psychotropic medication can differ between individuals. Having knowledge of the nuances between individual medications and how to respond to them is essential to medication management. Some medications have specific side effect profiles unique to them while others carry similar profiles within the broader groups. For example, selective serotonin reuptake inhibitors (SSRIs), a type of antidepressant, such as citalopram and fluoxetine, are not known to be sedating. However, sertraline, which is another SSRI in the same class, commonly causes drowsiness.

Another anti-depressant, mirtazapine, is sedating at lower doses, but this becomes less potent as the dose is increased. Knowledge of these side effects can support effective management of symptoms by using them for a therapeutic effect. For example, if someone is depressed and struggling to sleep, introducing a low dose of mirtazapine at night can be beneficial in improving sleep.

Activity 7.2 Reflection

Think of a time that you experienced side effects of medication.

- What was the medication and why were you taking it?
- What side effect did you experience? How did it make you feel?
- Did it change the way you feel about the medication that caused it? Or change the way you feel about medication in general?
- If you are asked to take the same medication again in the future, how would you respond?

Now consider the same questions in relation to when someone you were working with experienced side effects. And then consider:

- What did you do in that scenario?
- Is there anything you could have done differently to support that person?

As this activity is based on your own reflection, no outline answer is provided at the end of the chapter.

In subsequent sections of this chapter you will find a discussion of some of the most common side effects within the broad groups of psychotropic medication. It is not an exhaustive list and the use of clinical compendia or reference guides is helpful to clinical practice. The BNF (Joint Formulary Committee, 2021) gives more complete details of side effects and its app for smart phones and tablets is a useful tool for looking up potential side effects. There is also a function to check for interactions between medications, which is invaluable when working with people who take multiple medications.

Simple approaches to medication management, such as starting at a low dose and increasing slowly, can make all the difference to how severely individuals experience side effects. Those who are particularly sensitive to the side effects of medication can benefit from this approach, as it reduces the incidence of experiencing severe side effects on starting the medication. This approach works well in the case of anti-depressants and anxiolytics, where some of the more common side effects are more likely to occur at the start and sometimes improve with time. This way, nurses can support individuals to look out for signs of side effects and wait until that side effect resolves before an increased dose is considered, thus lessening the negative impact for the person on their experience of taking medication. With anti-psychotic medication, side effects are often dose-related and therefore starting at a lower dose and increasingly slowly means you can aim for the least amount of side effects and the best therapeutic response. Conversely, in the case of someone already experiencing unpleasant side effects from their anti-psychotic medication, a slight reduction in overall dose can sometimes lead to an improvement. The aim here is to use the smallest number of medications at the lowest effective dose. This can help reduce incidences of prescribing cascades, where someone is prescribed medication to alleviate the side effects of another.

When talking to people about the side effect experiences of the medication they are taking, it is important to remember that while many side effects are well known and attributed to certain medications, in the absence of any other explanation or cause, any reported effect should be considered as a potential side effect and reported through the yellow card system within the BNF. Taking these reports of side effects seriously will support a good working relationship between the individual and the nurse because they will feel listened to and taken seriously. This can improve the long-term health outcomes for the person for both their mental and physical health as well as their experiences of health care services.

That said, nurses must take care not to confuse side effects with discontinuation symptoms which occur when psychotropic medications are stopped abruptly. These symptoms are varied and can be mild effects such as headaches and sweating, up to more severe symptoms of agitation and delirium-like presentations. The risk of this is particularly high on admission to hospital and so the nurse has an important role to play in the reconciliation of medication.

Medication in older and younger population groups

In older adults, some anti-depressants, such as SSRIs, can increase the risk of bleeds and this must be considered as a potentially serious risk factor. Another type of anti-depressant, called tricyclics, can be toxic and tricyclics are much more likely to interact with other medications. This is important to remember as polypharmacy is common in this age group due to the multiple morbidities likely to occur. The rule of 'start low, go slow' is applied to this age group, which simply translates to starting at lower doses and increasing at slower rates in comparison to those for adults.

Older adults are likely to have reduced renal and liver functioning and, as most anti-psychotic medications are metabolised by the liver and excreted through the renal system, caution and monitoring of liver and renal functions may be prudent. Anti-psychotics can also lead to urinary retention and increase risk of falls, meaning extreme caution in this age group is advised. Older adults with Lewy body dementia and Parkinson's disease are prone to severe extrapyramidal side effects, a particular group of side effects seen in these medications, and therefore anti-psychotics are not recommended for this group of individuals.

For young people, anti-depressants are not licensed, indicated or recommended for treatment. This is partly because we have little knowledge of what impact they may have on brain development, and partly because clinical trials involving use of medication in children are difficult to conduct due to the myriad of legal and ethical implications. In extreme cases, the anti-depressant fluoxetine may be considered but should only be instigated by specialist secondary mental health services, never in primary care settings.

Anti-psychotic medications are also not licensed, indicated or recommended for treatment in under-18s. They are infrequently used in the case of severe mood disorders or in under-18s with learning difficulties when distress and/or aggression has not responded to all other interventions. In these cases, specialist services would be involved, and they should not be prescribed in primary care.

PART TWO

In Part Two we will look at some of the commonly seen groups of psychotropic medications seen in all areas of health care practice.

Anti-depressant medications

These groups of medications are used to treat a range of symptoms, and are therefore not exclusively seen in people experiencing a depressive disorder. They are commonly used in anxiety disorders such as generalised anxiety disorder, obsessive compulsive disorder and post-traumatic stress disorder. It is therefore important to be clear why they are being used for the individual.

Anti-depressants begin to work at the start of treatment; however the chemical changes required to elicit a therapeutic effect can take time. It is usual to see a therapeutic effect occur after 4–6 weeks for depressive symptoms and up to 12 weeks for anxiety symptoms. Informing people of the expectations of the drug and the response time can help to avoid disappointment and distress.

An indication of approximate recovery rates is shown in Figure 7.1. The 50% responding to first anti-depressant treatment may only see a reduction of their symptoms by around half (Taylor et al., 2021). This data reinforces the importance of trialling other interventions before considering an anti-depressant. Nurses can take an active role in ensuring that alternative psychosocial interventions such as reducing stress, improving diet and exercise and accessing talking therapies are used either before or alongside anti-depressant use.

It is thought that for those with moderate depression:

- 20% will recover with no treatment at all
- 30% will improve with placebo
- 50% will respond to first anti-depressant treatment (reduces with each anti-depressant thereafter if no response to the first)

(Anderson et al., 2008)

Figure 7.1 Approximate recovery rates with anti-depressants.

Anti-depressants are broadly grouped for their primary mode of action.

Selective serotonin reuptake inhibitors, commonly named SSRIs, block the reuptake of serotonin to increase the levels within the brain. They are 'selective' in that they focus on blocking the reuptake of the serotonin neurotransmitter 5-HT. Serotonin is linked to feelings of pleasure and contentment. Increased levels in the synaptic cleft can lead to an improvement in mood and a reduction in anxiety. However, it is important to be aware that an excess of serotonin can lead to a serious and potentially fatal condition called serotonin syndrome (Table 7.1). This can occur at any stage in the person's treatment and is not specific to SSRIs. Serotonin syndrome should be suspected in anyone taking an anti-depressant who presents with its signs and symptoms. This will require cessation of the anti-depressant and emergency care.

Symptoms of serotonin syndrome	Individuals at risk
Mild	
• Shivering • Diarrhoea • Confusion • Agitation • Fever • Muscle rigidity • Seizures	• Anyone taking an anti-depressant • Individuals taking more than one anti-depressant are at increased risk and this includes those switching from one to another • Individuals with a history of serotonin syndrome
Severe	

Table 7.1 Serotonin syndrome

Serotonin noradrenaline reuptake inhibitors, or SNRIs, act in a similar way to SSRIs but block the reuptake of both serotonin and noradrenaline. They tend to be second-line options for those who have not responded to SSRIs and come with a similar side effect profile.

Tricyclic anti-depressants are a second- or third-line treatment option for those not responding to SSRIs/SNRIs. Tricyclics prevent reabsorption of noradrenaline and serotonin into the nerve cells and are not selective in their action. Consequently, they have more unpleasant side effects and are cardiotoxic and dangerous in overdose. This means caution is required in individuals who are at risk of overdose.

Monoamine oxidase inhibitors, or MAOIs, are rarely seen in contemporary mental health care. However, if someone is prescribed these medications it is important to be aware that certain foods should not be consumed. This is because MAOIs inhibit the enzyme monoamine oxidase, which is used to break down excess levels of the amino acid, tyramine. If the body's ability to break down excess tyramine is impaired, it can lead to hypertensive crisis and death. Therefore, foods with high levels of tyramine should not be consumed. This includes foods that have been fermented, cured or aged, and some beans and overripe fruits.

Other anti-depressants, such as mirtazapine and trazodone, are chemically different but produce similar effects (Table 7.2). They tend to be sedating and therefore helpful when given at night to aid sleep; however the sedating effect can interfere with people's ability to perform skilled tasks the next day. Mirtazapine acts in a way that means it is more sedating at lower doses but with a better anti-depressant effect at higher doses. Consequently, it is often used alongside another anti-depressant to aid sleep while the other is used to treat the depressive symptoms.

Types	Examples	Indications	Common side effects	Special considerations
SSRIs and SNRIs	SSRIs: Sertraline Citalopram Fluoxetine SNRIs: Venlafaxine Duloxetine	Depressive illness, major depression, obsessive compulsive disorder, panic disorder, post-traumatic stress disorder, social anxiety disorder, generalised anxiety disorder	Anxiety, arrhythmia, asthenia, impaired concentration, confusion, constipation, depersonalisation, diarrhoea, dizziness, dry mouth, fever, gastrointestinal discomfort, headache, irregular menstrual cycle, myalgia, nausea (dose-related), QT interval prolongation, sexual dysfunction, altered taste, tinnitus, weight changes	Risk of developing serotonin syndrome with all anti-depressants. Fluoxetine has a longer half-life and is first choice in under-18s or in pregnancy. With some SNRIs, the side effect of sexual dysfunction may persist after treatment is stopped
Tricyclics	Imipramine Trimipramine Clomipramine	Depressive illness, phobic and obsessional states, major depressive disorder	Anxiety, arrhythmia, cardiac conduction disorders, confusion, delirium, drowsiness, dizziness, epilepsy, hallucinations, headache, hepatic disorders, palpitations, sexual dysfunction, skin reactions, weight changes	Toxic in overdose. Trimipramine is indicated where sedation is required. Amitriptyline is not recommended in depressive illness due to risk of fatality in overdose

(Continued)

Table 7.2   (Continued)

Types	Examples	Indications	Common side effects	Special considerations
Other anti-depressants	Mirtazapine Trazodone Reboxetine	Major depression, anxiety	Anxiety, arthralgia, back pain, confusion, akathisia, constipation, diarrhoea, dizziness, drowsiness, dry mouth, myalgia, nausea, oedema, hyperhidrosis, postural hypotension, sleep disorders, tremor, vomiting, weight increased, agranulocytosis, blood disorders, gastrointestinal discomfort, reduced libido, thrombocytopenia, vertigo	Mirtazapine can aid sleep so may be first-line choice in some cases. Trazodone may be indicated where sedation is required

Table 7.2   Commonly used medications: anti-depressants

SSRIs, selective serotonin reuptake inhibitors; SNRIs, serotonin noradrenaline reuptake inhibitors

Anti-psychotic medication

These medications are again grouped for their mode of action into typical and atypical anti-psychotics and are used for a variety of symptoms. Their primary use is for the treatment of psychosis; however it is not uncommon in practice to see them used in mood-related disorders such as bipolar affective disorder or even to alleviate some of the symptoms of personality disorders. Similarly, low doses can be used to treat symptoms of anxiety or post-traumatic stress disorder. As discussed earlier in the chapter, the use of medications in any scenario should not be first-line and this applies to anti-psychotic medication. The potential for cardiac effects along with drug interactions and unwanted side effects can make them undesirable for individuals to take. Close monitoring and management of the effects are important to optimise outcomes. The annual monitoring requirements for these medications are listed in Figure 7.2.

- Blood test – FBC, LFT, renal, fasting lipids (HDL/LDL), glucose/HbA1c
- Blood pressure and pulse
- ECG
- Waist circumference and body mass index
- Record smoking status, and provide lifestyle advice on smoking, alcohol intake, diet and exercise

Figure 7.2   Annual care requirements for individuals taking anti-psychotic medication. FBC, full blood count; LFT, liver function tests; HDL, high-density lipoprotein; LDL, low-density lipoprotein; ECG, electrocardiogram.

Some anti-psychotics come in injectable forms such as fast-acting or long-acting depot preparations. Liquids and soluble oral tablets are also available. This versatility in preparation is helpful in circumstances where treatment is being carefully monitored, there are serious implications of missed doses, when enforced treatment is required or according to personal preference.

High-dose anti-psychotic treatment (HDAT) is a term used to identify those individuals taking greater than 100% maximum doses of anti-psychotics. This increases the risks of adverse effects and requires increased monitoring. It occurs rarely in planned treatment regimes. In practice environments, an individual can be put at risk through HDAT if their acute presentation of psychosis, agitation or aggression is treated with as required anti-psychotics alongside their regular anti-psychotic medication. For example, someone taking 20 mg olanzapine daily is already on 100% of the maximum dose. If they are then given a further 5 mg as required for agitation, which is 25% of the maximum dose, this gives them a total of 125% of olanzapine and is classed as HDAT. The same principle applies if someone is given two different anti-psychotics concurrently. Therefore, it is important for nurses to be aware of maximum doses, working out the percentage given and ensuring this does not total more than 100%.

Each anti-psychotic has its own side effect profile and therefore it is important to review their individual effects. Olanzapine, for example, is an atypical anti-psychotic known to cause weight gain, hyperglycaemia, oedema and sedation. In contrast, risperidone, also an atypical anti-psychotic, is more likely to cause gynaecomastia, hyperprolactinaemia and sexual dysfunction. As a rule, taking any anti-psychotics can result in having these side effects. However, some have more moderate effects than others. In practice, taking one with a lower capacity for weight gain may be favourable for someone with type 2 diabetes, where the benefits outweigh the risk of side effects.

Neuroleptic malignant syndrome is a serious and potentially fatal adverse effect of anti-psychotic medication (Table 7.3). The risk is slightly higher with typical anti-psychotics

Signs of neuroleptic malignant syndrome	Individuals at risk
• Confusion • Agitation • Delirium • Fever / pyrexia • Irregular pulse • Variable blood pressure • Tachypnoea • Muscle rigidity and/or tremor • Raised creatinine phosphokinase • seizures	• Anyone taking an anti-psychotic at any point in their treatment • Individuals having high-dose anti-psychotic treatment (HDAT) • Individuals with a history of neuroleptic malignant syndrome

Table 7.3   Neuroleptic malignant syndrome

but should be considered for anyone presenting with its signs and symptoms and taking any anti-psychotic medication.

Raised levels of prolactin are not uncommon and can often lead to galactorrhoea and gynaecomastia, which are both distressing for the individual and can also indicate an impact on fertility and sexual functioning. Metabolic syndrome is a group of risk factors associated with cardiovascular disease and diabetes and increases the risk of health complications such as stroke. The risk factors involved are:

- elevated waist circumference;
- raised blood pressure (or drug treatment for hypertension);
- raised fasting blood glucose (or drug treatment for hyperglycaemia);
- elevated triglycerides;
- low levels of high-density lipid (cholesterol).

The presence of three out of five of these factors would constitute a diagnosis of metabolic syndrome. Annual monitoring and advice on lifestyle can help identify risk factors early and provide opportunities for health promotion.

Anti-psychotic medications are broadly grouped into typical and atypical anti-psychotics (Table 7.4):

- *Typical anti-psychotics*, also known as first-generation, were largely developed in the 1950s and 1960s. They block dopamine D_2 receptor sites, leading to a decrease in dopaminergic activity in the brain. These anti-psychotics bring the risk of a specific group of side effects called extrapyramidal side effects (EPSEs). These include hypersalivation, motor rigidity, tardive dyskinesia, dystonia and shuffling gait. It is useful to monitor these before and during treatment.
- *Atypical anti-psychotics*, also known as second-generation, came later and were thought to have less severe side effects than their predecessors. They influence both dopamine and serotonin 5-HT receptors and transporters. Most common side effects are metabolic, such as weight gain, sedation and raised prolactin.
- *Clozapine* is a second-generation anti-psychotic medication. As a result of cases of sudden death following its original introduction in the 1960s, there are strict protocols around its use. It was later reintroduced, with a national Clozapine Patient Monitoring Service (CPMS) to regulate its use and supply and to monitor blood results to ensure individuals are not developing signs of neutropenia and agranulocytosis. These can be severe and fatal side effects of the drug. Pre-treatment requirements include a blood test and electrocardiogram. Doses are started from 12.5 mg and titrated upwards. Missed doses of more than 48 hours will need to be retitrated from a starting dose. Abrupt cessation can cause rebound psychosis, agitation, catatonia and cholinergic rebound. Liaising with mental health teams for advice and guidance around clozapine is essential due to its complicated nature and strict regulations.

Types	Examples	Indications	Common side effects	Special considerations
Typical / first-generation Atypical / second-generation	Typical: Haloperidol Zuclopenthixol Flupentixol Trifluoperazine Atypical: Olanzapine Quetiapine Risperidone Aripiprazole	Schizophrenia, schizoaffective disorder, delirium, mania associated with bipolar disorder, acute agitation, persistent aggression in dementia (haloperidol), acute and chronic psychosis, preventing recurrence of bipolar disorder, agitation in mania or psychosis, adjunct in treatment of depression (quetiapine)	EPSEs such as dystonia, akathisia, QT interval prolongation, arrhythmias, tremor, insomnia, weight gain, insulin resistance, sexual dysfunction, amenorrhoea, drowsiness, dry mouth, galactorrhoea, gynaecomastia, hyperprolactinaemia, urinary retention	Dystonia common in young males who are neuroleptic-naive. Annual monitoring required to prevent risk factors associated with metabolic syndrome
Clozapine (second-generation)	Clozapine	Schizophrenia where no response to at least two other anti-psychotics. Titration starting at 12.5 mg up to max. 900 mg daily	Same as first- and second-generation plus: severe constipation and peristalsis, neutropenia, agranulocytosis, seizures, myocarditis, cardiomyopathy	Registration with a Patient Monitoring Service required. Pre-treatment blood test and ECG needed. During treatment, weekly, fortnightly or monthly blood test required. Must be re-titrated if doses missed for more than 48 hours

Table 7.4 Commonly used medications: anti-psychotics

EPSE, extrapyramidal side effects; ECG, electrocardiogram.

Mood-stabilising medication

The term 'mood stabiliser' is used to denote medications that are used to prevent recurrent depressive episodes, mania or a mixed affective state seen in bipolar affective disorder or schizoaffective disorder.

Depression is the predominant mood state in bipolar affective disorders. Research suggests that anywhere between 67% and 94% of symptomatic individuals with a diagnosis of bipolar affective disorder will be depressed (Judd et al., 2002, 2003). The so-called 'mixed state' in mood disorders, where an individual will experience symptoms of both low and elevated mood at the same time, occurs at a similar frequency to that of mania. Because of the nature of these fluctuating mood states, treatment with both mood stabilisers and anti-depressants may be indicated in these instances.

Very few mood stabilisers are effective in preventing both high and low mood states. Therefore, a combination of medications is often used to treat or at least reduce the frequency and severity of episodes. This is not without risks as anti-depressants used to prevent depression can induce mania. Therefore, stopping anti-depressant treatment in anyone presenting with symptoms of mania should be considered. This decision should not be taken lightly as it can increase the risk of a potential depressive episode following the period of mania. And rapid withdrawal can be very unpleasant for the individual. Some anti-psychotic medications have been found to be beneficial, particularly in acute phases of mania. They are therefore commonly used as an alternative or alongside a mood stabiliser or anti-depressant.

Commonly used mood stabilisers and their properties are as follows:

Lithium carbonate and lithium citrate are lithium salts with similar chemical properties to sodium. Their exact mechanism is difficult to ascertain. It can be effective in the treatment of mania. Because it takes time for serum lithium levels to reach optimal levels, an anti-psychotic medication is sometimes used alongside lithium in the early stages of treatment. Lithium has been found to be effective, and superior to anti-depressants, in preventing relapses of low mood associated with bipolar disorder (Cipriani et al., 2006). Lithium is excreted through the renal system and is therefore not recommended for those with renal impairment.

Monitoring of serum lithium levels is an essential part of treatment. The optimum serum level is 0.4–1.0 mmol/L. For prevention of recurrent mania, a serum level of 0.7–1.0 mmol/L is advised. Blood samples must be taken at least 12 hours after dose for optimum readings. This is done 5–7 days after commencing treatment or any dose changes, then a minimum of every 3 months, throughout treatment, once the dose and serum levels are stable in the optimum range.

Lithium toxicity occurs when the serum lithium level becomes too high or when the body is unable to metabolise and excrete lithium effectively (Table 7.5).

Signs of lithium toxicity	Risk factors	Management
• Confusion • Slurred speech • Tremor • Unstable blood pressure • Pyrexia • Muscle weakness • Diarrhoea • Vomiting • Seizures • Death	• Anyone taking lithium • Those with poor renal function • Can occur at any stage in treatment	• Stop lithium immediately and seek medical advice • Lithium levels should be taken as soon as possible and liver and renal function should be checked • In the event of severe toxicity, emergency response and admission to an acute hospital are required

Table 7.5 Lithium toxicity

This serious and potentially fatal complication makes it essential that anyone taking lithium or considering it as a treatment option is aware of this risk. It is vital that nurses are aware of the signs of toxicity and can respond accordingly. Lithium toxicity will always lead to the cessation of lithium, even if only for a short period. With mildly elevated levels in healthy adults showing no signs of toxicity, it is possible that missing one or two doses is enough to reduce the level and restart the lithium, possibly at a lower dose.

- *Sodium valproate,* an anti-convulsant, has also been successful in treating bipolar affective disorder. It has become a widely accepted treatment alternative to lithium for mood disorders despite being unlicensed. There are now strict protocols around its use in women of childbearing age because of known complications in pregnancy.
- *Lamotrigine* is another anti-convulsant effective in preventing, or reducing the severity and frequency of, recurrent periods of low mood (Table 7.6). It is rarely used in acute treatment because it requires a slow upward dose titration. However, it is sometimes commenced in the acute phase with long-term prophylaxis in mind.

Mood stabiliser	Indication	Common side effects	Special considerations
Lithium salts (citrate and carbonate)	Treatment and prophylaxis of mania, bipolar disorder, recurrent depression Treatment and prophylaxis of aggressive or self-harming behaviour	Dizziness, dry mouth, tremor, electrolyte imbalance, hypotension, cardiomyopathy, atrioventricular block. Arrhythmias, hypothyroidism, hyperparathyroidism, nystagmus, renal impairment, seizure, thyrotoxicosis, vision impairment	Therapeutic level 0.4–1 mmol/L. Risk of toxicity at any stage in treatment. Long-term use associated with thyroid disorder and mild cognitive impairment. Adjusted doses and increased monitoring required in renal impairment
Lamotrigine	Monotherapy or adjunctive therapy with or without sodium valproate for bipolar disorder	Agitation, arthralgia, diarrhoea, dizziness, drowsiness, dry mouth, fatigue, headache, nausea, pain, rash, tremor. Stevens–Johnson syndrome and other serious skin conditions can also occur	Dose adjustment required when used with enzyme-inducing drugs or with hepatic impairment
Sodium valproate	Mania Unlicensed use: Treatment and prophylaxis of bipolar disorder	Abdominal pain, agitation, alopecia, anaemia, impaired concentration, confusion, diarrhoea, drowsiness, hepatic disorders, hyponatraemia, memory loss, nystagmus, tremor, urinary disorders, weight gain	Not to be used in women of childbearing age without robust contraceptive plans. Monitoring of liver function before and after 6 months is required

Table 7.6 Commonly used medications: mood stabilisers

Anxiolytic medication

Anxiety is a normal human emotion. Health care professionals need to be able to distinguish between normal anxiety and anxiety that is part of a mental illness. It is normal to feel anxious, overwhelmed or out of control in scenarios such as starting a new job, examinations, deadlines during court proceedings or because of a loss, bereavement or traumatic event. In these cases, the individual is likely to respond to brief psychosocial or psychological interventions.

In anxiety disorders such as generalised anxiety disorder, obsessive compulsive disorder or post-traumatic stress disorder, anxiety is the underlying theme but presents with a range of other signs and symptoms. Medication may be indicated when there are concerns for the safety of the person or those around them, where there is a significant impact on functioning or where there has been no response to psychological or psychosocial interventions.

Anti-depressants, specifically SSRIs and SNRIs, are the preferred choice. These can initially exacerbate anxiety and therefore lower starting doses are recommended. Although this effect is likely to improve after the first few days, informing individuals about it is helpful. This can be seen in the following case study where Amir, who was introduced in Part One, returns to see his practice nurse for another asthma review.

Case study: revisiting Amir

Amir (25) returns to see his practice nurse for an asthma review. His asthma is well controlled, but he confides that his anxiety is still a problem and seems to be getting worse.

Since his last visit, he has completed a course of CBT which has given him some tools to manage day to day. He thinks these tools are useful, but he has noticed that things are getting progressively worse. He is no longer socialising with friends as this tends to provoke panic attacks. Some mornings he is too anxious to leave the house and he is at risk of losing his job due to repeated episodes of sickness.

The nurse suggests Amir arranges to see his general practitioner (GP) to discuss other treatment options. The GP gathers the history and considers that the use of medication is indicated at this stage due to the impact of Amir's anxiety on his functioning and quality of life. They discuss the option of trialling an SSRI anti-depressant. Amir is given information on several of these first-line medications so he can weigh up the pros and cons and make an informed decision about whether he wishes to try them.

The GP is careful to explain the potential for an initial worsening of his anxiety and suggests Amir starts this new medication during his upcoming annual leave to lessen the chance of further absence from work in the initial stages or treatment.

Medications used in the long-term management of anxiety disorders are as follows (Table 7.7):

- *Anti-depressants,* specifically SSRIs and SNRIs, are the preferred choice. All have the potential to worsen anxiety initially and are therefore started at lower doses in comparison to those used for depression. The tricyclic anti-depressant clomipramine can be useful in generalised anxiety disorder and obsessive compulsive disorder.
- *Anti-psychotic medication,* such as the atypical anti-psychotic quetiapine, has been shown to have some impact on anxiety, albeit in lower doses than would be seen for psychosis or mood-related illness.
- *Beta-blockers,* such as propranolol, are often effective in panic disorder to reduce the impact of the physiological symptoms triggered in the autonomic nervous system which are responsible for high levels of distress to the individual. They are contraindicated in asthma.
- *Pregabalin* is an anti-convulsant and gamma-aminobutyric acid (GABA) analogue which is licensed for the treatment of generalised anxiety disorder. The effects are rapid, but tolerability of side effects varies. Stopping pregabalin abruptly can lead to seizures. Misuse of pregabalin is common and it is an offence to be in its possession without a prescription. Individuals should be informed of this prior to commencing treatment.
- *Benzodiazepines* are effective anxiolytics but are recommended for short-term use only because of the potential to develop tolerance and dependence with continued use. Even in the short term, they should be used with caution as their ability to rapidly reduce an individual's anxiety levels can lead to a natural desire to use them repeatedly, rather than develop important psychological strategies to support long-term recovery.

Anxiolytic medication	Indication	Common side effects	Special considerations
Clomipramine (tricyclic anti-depressant)	Depression, phobias, obsessive thinking	Anxiety, arrhythmia, breast enlargement, constipation, diarrhoea, fatigue, hypotension, confusion, dry mouth, hot flush, drowsiness and dizziness, headaches, QT prolongation	Clomipramine increased the effects of adrenaline/ epinephrine. Withdrawal symptoms on cessation common
Pregabalin (anti-convulsant)	Generalised anxiety disorder	Abdominal distension, constipation, impaired concentration, confusion, drowsiness, dry mouth, memory loss, nausea, oedema, respiratory depression	Risk of abuse and dependence. Abrupt withdrawal can precipitate seizures
Propranolol (beta-blocker)	Physiological effects of anxiety (palpitations, sweating, tremor, etc.)	Bradycardia, confusion, depression, dizziness, dry eye, dyspnoea, erectile dysfunction, paraesthesia, peripheral coldness, syncope	Exacerbates asthma. Risks in pregnancy and breastfeeding

Table 7.7 Commonly used medications: anxiolytics

Anti-dementia medication

'Dementia' is an umbrella term used to denote a group of diagnoses associated with a decline in brain functioning. It encompasses Alzheimer's disease, vascular dementia, Lewy body dementia and cognitive impairment, among others. Before a diagnosis of dementia can be made, physical health screening is required to rule out common differential diagnoses. Infection, stroke, atrial fibrillation, hypo- and hyperthyroidism as well as delirium are some examples of physical health problems that can present like dementia (Holland, 2018).

Treatment options are limited. The aim of anti-dementia medication is to slow down the progression of the illness, but it cannot stop it entirely. Shared decision making is important to help the person and their loved ones decide whether medication is the best course of action. Medication is not the only option as many symptoms of dementia can be managed with environmental or psychosocial interventions.

The neurotransmitter acetylcholine is believed to play a role in memory and learning as well as the regulation of mood and behaviour. Decreased levels are therefore thought to be a contributing factor in dementia. Most anti-dementia medications are designed to inhibit the enzyme that breaks down acetylcholine.

Medications used to slow the progression of dementia include the following (Table 7.8):

- *Anti-cholinesterase inhibitors* inhibit the action of acetylcholinesterase, an enzyme that breaks down acetylcholine. This leads to an increase of acetylcholine in the brain. The anti-cholinesterase inhibitors available are rivastigmine, donepezil and galantamine.
- The *N-methyl-D-aspartate (NMDA) receptor antagonist*, memantine, acts as an antagonist at the NMDA receptor and protects the brain from excess glutamate that is produced because of the damage caused by Alzheimer's disease.

Anti-dementia medication	Indication and dose	Common side effects	Special considerations
Anti-cholinesterase inhibitors: Rivastigmine Donepezil Galantamine	Mild to moderately severe dementia in Alzheimer's disease	Dizziness, nausea, diarrhoea, urinary incontinence, arrhythmia, fatigue, insomnia, agitation, tremor, bradycardia, atrioventricular block, seizures, gastric ulcers	Rivastigmine also used for dementia in Parkinson's disease
N-methyl-D-aspartate (NMDA) receptor antagonist: Memantine	Moderate to severe dementia in Alzheimer's disease	Impaired balance, constipation, drowsiness, dizziness, headache, hypertension, difficulty breathing. Embolism and thrombosis (rarely)	Also used for oscillopsia in multiple sclerosis

Table 7.8 Commonly used medications: anti-dementia

Short-term medication for acute problems

Some symptoms associated with mental health problems are not unique to any one diagnosis but may need treatment with medication in acute phases (Table 7.9).

Medication	Indication	Common side effects	Special considerations
Lorazepam Clonazepam Diazepam (benzodiazepines)	Short-term use in anxiety or insomnia, acute panic attacks, acute agitation (such as catatonia), panic disorders resistant to anti-depressant treatment	Reduced alertness, ataxia, confusion, dizziness, drowsiness, dysarthria, fatigue, gastrointestinal disorder, headache, muscle weakness, nausea, hypotension, vertigo, respiratory depression (especially in overdose)	Only for short-term use due to risk of abuse and dependence. In the case of dependence, switch to a long-acting benzodiazepine and slowly reduce dose every 2–4 weeks
'Z drugs': Zopiclone Zolpidem	Insomnia (short-term use)	Dry mouth, bitter taste, anxiety, dizziness, fatigue, headache, confusion and impaired concentration, anterograde amnesia	Risk of tolerance and withdrawals. Caution in older adults. Reduced doses in hepatic and renal impairment
Melatonin	Insomnia (short-term use)	Arthralgia, headaches, increased risk of infection, anxiety, dizziness, dry mouth, night sweats, nausea	Not licensed for use in those with learning disabilities
Promethazine	Sedation (short-term use)	Arrhythmia, confusion, dizziness, dry mouth, headache, blurred vision, agranulocytosis, angle closure glaucoma, anticholinergic syndrome, nausea, rash, seizure	Older adults particularly susceptible to anti-cholinergic side effects

Table 7.9 Commonly used medications: acute problems

Insomnia is common in all mental illness. Starting medication for the underlying problem is beneficial for long-term recovery but use of short-term benzodiazepines or hypnotics can also be helpful. In many cases, this will be where sleep hygiene interventions have failed, or the effects of impaired sleep are preventing recovery or having a prolonged negative impact on functioning.

Agitation often occurs in acute phases and is important to treat, particularly if the individual is highly distressed. Although some forms of agitation are evident through an individual's behaviour, some is internalised and more difficult to identify. Someone with an agitated or psychotic a depressive disorder, for example, may present with an inability to articulate their thoughts, sweating, rubbing of their forehead, pained expressions, continually ruminating and being 'stuck' on a topic or problem. Although the person is not aggressive or overactive, there could be a high level of internal agitation which can significantly impair their functioning.

Catatonia is common in acute and severe episodes of both psychotic illnesses such as schizophrenia and schizoaffective disorders and, somewhat less commonly, in bipolar mood disorders. Here, an individual can oscillate between long periods of inactivity, severe motor retardation and acute episodes of extreme activity such as running up and down the room. Small doses of benzodiazepines can reduce agitation enough for the person to think, feel and behave more clearly.

Rapid tranquillisation

In extreme situations, when all else has failed, it may be necessary to use rapid tranquil-lisation. This is medication given in an emergency to reduce agitation and aggression caused by mental illness. NICE defines rapid tranquillisation as:

> *the use of medication by the parenteral route (usually intramuscular or, exceptionally, intravenous) if oral medication is not possible or appropriate and urgent sedation with medication is needed* (NICE, 2015, page 19).

The intention should be to calm or lightly sedate the person. This form of treatment is used as a last resort and would only be expected to take place in hospital settings.

Before rapid tranquillisation, it is important to consider other factors at play. This could include existing physical health problems, possible intoxication, pregnancy, current medications and the potential for interactions, and previous response to medications used in rapid tranquillisation. Existing knowledge of the person's preference, advance statements and decisions is also a vital consideration in these situations.

After rapid tranquillisation is administered, the person should be closely monitored for therapeutic response, adverse effects and signs of physical deterioration. Respiratory depression is associated with this type of administration along with side effects of the individual medicines used, such as neuroleptic malignant syndrome or the cardiac effects associated with anti-psychotic medication such as arrhythmias, hypertension, orthostatic hypotension and myocarditis. National guidelines suggest monitoring the person's pulse, blood pressure, respiratory rate, temperature, level of consciousness along with fluid input and output at least every hour, or every 15 minutes in the event that high doses have been given, the person is intoxicated with drugs or alcohol or in the presence of pre-existing physical health problems. Many mental health trusts will monitor vital signs every 15 minutes for 1 hour, every hour for 2 hours, every 2 hours for 12 hours and every 4 hours for 24 hours following rapid tranquillisation.

Post-incident debriefs for the health care professionals involved and the individual them-selves are also important. The purpose of the conversation with the individual is to talk to them about what happened, hear their reflections on the event, explain why rapid tran-quillisation was felt to be needed and consider what actions could be taken to avoid the situation in the future. This is a joint conversation that requires active involvement from both parties and should be approached from a non-judgemental position by the nurse.

Rapid tranquillisation in children and young people is rare; however separate guidance is provided by the Paediatric Innovation, Education and Research (PIER) Network in their *Rapid Tranquillisation and the Management of Violent and Aggressive Paediatric Patients* guidelines (Hill et al., 2018). This is a helpful resource in inpatient areas where nurses are working with highly distressed young people.

Choosing medication for the purpose of rapid tranquillisation

NICE has published guidance on the use of rapid tranquillisation within its *Violence and Aggression: Short-Term Management in Mental Health, Health and Community Settings* document (NICE, 2015) (Figure 7.3).

---

1. If there is insufficient information to guide the choice of medication for rapid tranquillisation, or the service user has not taken antipsychotic medication before, use intramuscular lorazepam
2. If there is evidence of cardiovascular disease, including a prolonged QT interval, or no electrocardiogram has been carried out, use intramuscular lorazepam instead. Intramuscular haloperidol with or without intramuscular promethazine should be avoided
3. If there is a partial response to intramuscular lorazepam, consider a further dose
4. If there is no response to intramuscular lorazepam, consider intramuscular haloperidol either alone or combined with intramuscular promethazine
5. If there is a partial response to intramuscular haloperidol combined with intramuscular promethazine, consider a further dose

---

Figure 7.3 A stepped approach to rapid tranquillisation (adapted from NICE, 2015).

Chapter summary

In this chapter, we have looked at medication used to alleviate the symptoms of mental illness and considered the implications for practice. This includes the potential benefits and limitations of medication, as well as the importance of using other interventions either instead of, or alongside, medication. Ensuring shared decision making is essential to enhancing the outcomes of the individuals in our care.

The landscape of medication use in mental health is ever changing and research continues with emerging evidence around the use of amphetamines, hallucinogens and cannabis to alleviate symptoms of mental illness. Regardless of the chemical being used, there will always be limitations and so the role of the nurse is to educate, advise and support the individual to make informed decisions wherever possible.

Activities: Brief outline answers

Activity 7.1 Reflection (page 112)

Here are some ways in which you can ensure you respond to the patients' mental health needs alongside their physical health:

- *Ask questions:* having an open and enquiring stance can be helpful in gaining information on people's mental health and any medication they are taking.
- *Listen to what the person is saying:* hearing and acknowledging people's experience of medication is powerful and can make them feel heard and cared for.
- *Respond to their wants and needs:* suggesting simple solutions such as talking to their GP or mental health team about their medication or getting advice from mental health liaison teams in hospital settings can be the first step towards improving the person's experience of medication.
- *Play to their strengths:* suggest alternatives to help support their mental health outside of using medication by identifying their strengths or hobbies and using those to improve their wellbeing.
- *Look for other solutions:* don't assume medication is the answer. Many people don't want it and may not even need it. Consider psychosocial interventions such as education, self-help and social prescribing.

All these brief and simple interventions, along with many more, can be applied in all health care settings. One brief intervention can make such a difference and can often be achieved in just a few short minutes.

Further reading

Rogers, J, Leung, C and Nicholson, T (2020) *British Association for Psychopharmacology Pocket Prescriber Psychiatry.* London: CRC Press.

Gives succinct information on pharmacological properties and considerations for practice.

Taylor, D, Barnes, T, and Young, A (2021) *The Maudsley Prescribing Guidelines in Psychiatry* (14th edition). Oxford: Wiley-Blackwell.

Draws on the best evidence base to support prescribing.

The Joint Formulary Committee (2021) *The British National Formulary.* Available online at: https://bnf.nice.org.uk/

Produced in print as well as electronic forms and the BNF app for smartphones and tablets.

Chapter 8 Managing stress and promoting your mental health

Steve Trenoweth and Chloe Casey

NMC Future Nurse: Standards of Proficiency for Registered Nurses

This chapter will address the following platforms and proficiencies:

Platform 1: Being an accountable professional

At the point of registration, the registered nurse will be able to:

1.5 understand the demands of professional practice and demonstrate how to recognise signs of vulnerability in themselves or their colleagues and the action required to minimise risks to health.

1.6 understand the professional responsibility to adopt a healthy lifestyle to maintain the level of personal fitness and wellbeing required to meet people's needs for mental and physical care.

1.10 demonstrate resilience and emotional intelligence and be capable of explaining the rationale that influences their judgments and decisions in routine, complex and challenging situations.

1.17 take responsibility for continuous self-reflection, seeking and responding to support and feedback to develop their professional knowledge and skills.

1.19 act as an ambassador, upholding the reputation of their profession and promoting public confidence in nursing, health and care services.

Chapter aims

After reading this chapter, you will be able to:

- understand the different types of stress we may experience, its effects on us and what we can do about it;
- understand adaptive and maladaptive coping;

(Continued)

(Continued)

- develop your own stress management toolkit;
- understand how nursing students can develop their own coping styles whilst adopting a mentally healthy lifestyle.

Introduction

Stress is sadly all too common in health services and amongst nursing staff. In this chapter, readers are invited to consider their own mental health and how this may be developed and enhanced to support their own wellbeing and the delivery of nursing care. Those of us who work in health care are often exposed to work-related stress due to the nature of our roles and work context (such as busy clinical and nursing environments, the emotional burden of caring, burnout, pressured life-or-death decisions). But, of course, nurses and other health care practitioners are exposed to the same stressors as the general population.

In this chapter, we start by looking at stress, the different types of stress we may experience, its effects on us and what we can do about it. The notion of adaptive and maladaptive coping will be explored along with how we can develop our own stress management toolkit. The issue of resilience is one that features in the new nursing curricula, along with how nursing students can develop their own coping styles whilst adopting a mentally healthy lifestyle.

What is stress?

Stress is very common. It is also pervasive in that it can affect all aspects of our lives and can have a significant impact on our physical and mental health and wellbeing. While we cannot always avoid stress in our lives, there are many ways in which we can learn to cope with stress, thereby moderating its detrimental effects on us.

Stress is an anxious emotional state. It is triggered by perceived threats or fear. Stress tests our coping abilities and is a significant health problem for individuals, employers and society. According to Richard Lazarus (1999), we become stressed when events and responsibilities exceed our ability to cope with them. When we perceive a threat, our body undergoes complex physiological processes to ensure that we are prepared to respond – that is, to fight the threat or to flee (van der Kolk, 2014). Stress is, therefore, a normal human response to threats that we perceive in our environment and can be helpful to our survival. However, stress can become a problem when we feel overwhelmed by a *stressor* and/or we feel unable to respond to a perceived threat.

Types of stress

There are different ways of conceptualising stress (Table 8.1).

Acute stress	Acute stress is intense in nature but short in duration. This is known as the *freeze, fight or flight* response – the body's physiological arousal to respond to or survive a threat. The body prepares itself (by release of hormones) to fight/defend itself from a threat or run and escape the danger. This can be triggered by real or imaginary threats. However, we no longer face the sorts of threats to our survival that our bodies have been evolutionarily prepared for. That is, our body does not distinguish between being attacked by a bear and receiving a bill we can't pay: they are both perceived as threats.
Chronic stress	Chronic stress is not as intense as acute stress but lingers for a prolonged period of time. This places our bodies at serious risk of poor health.
Eustress	This is any stressor which is ultimately helpful. The Yerkes–Dodson (1908) principle states that *eustress*, in *optimal* doses, can motivate us to improve our physical performance and our thinking and concentration.

Table 8.1 Types of stress

Broadly speaking, there are two types of stress that we may experience in our lives: *background stress* (or daily hassles) and *life event stress*. Let's have a look at these.

Background stress (daily hassles)

Our background stress arises from daily hassles (Kanner et al., 1981) – those frequent irritating, frustrating, distressing demands or practical difficulties which are part of our daily lives. This type of stress comes from a number of sources:

- *social hassles* (e.g. crowding, queuing, being ignored or talked over, experiencing discrimination);
- *interpersonal hassles* (e.g. family problems, conflict, arguments);
- *situational hassles* (e.g. traffic jams);
- *practical hassles* (e.g. accommodation problems, bills, debt, rising costs, misplacing or losing things);
- *health-related hassles* (e.g. hassles arising from personal health, long-term conditions or health of a family member, caring responsibilities);
- *environmental hassles* (e.g. noise, pollution, living in an overcrowded area, high crime rates);
- *technological hassles* (e.g. information overload, being too available, too many interruptions);
- *work-related stress* (e.g. being unhappy at work, having too many responsibilities, obligations and things to do, not having enough time, threat of redundancy or changes to working conditions).

The impact of daily hassles on our health is affected by:

- the *number* of daily hassles we experience;
- the *repetition* and *frequency* of hassles;
- the *compounding effect* of daily hassles during a rare life event or a crisis;
- our ability (or inability) to *cope* and *manage* daily hassles.

Work-related stress can be a significant source of background stress. The Health and Safety Executive (HSE) (2019) noted that sources of work-related stress can arise from our experience of:

- *excessive demands and workload* (work patterns and the working environment);
- *poor control over our work* (how much say the person has in the way they do their work);
- *limited encouragement and support* (sponsorship and resources provided by the organisation, line management and colleagues);
- *damaged interpersonal relationships at work* (promoting positive working practices to avoid conflict and dealing with unacceptable behaviour);
- *poor understanding of role* (and/or having conflicting roles);
- *poor management of change* (how organisational change (large or small) is managed and communicated in the organisation);
- *organisational culture* (the way in which organisations demonstrate management commitment and have procedures which are fair and open).

So, while each daily hassle may be relatively minor in itself, they may *accumulate* (build up and multiply) and become *amplified*, making them more significant (for example, ongoing conflict and arguments with our partners may lead to us being less able to cope with minor disagreements at work).

Activity 8.1   Reflection

Take some time to review the material in this section and start to compile a list of your daily hassles and work stressors. How might you manage these stressors and the impact they have on your life?

As this activity is based on your own reflection, no outline answer is provided at the end of the chapter.

Life event stress

For Holmes and Rahe (1967), many life events represent a psychological crisis for us (they catalogued 43 such significant life crises). They saw these crises as being rare, sometimes life-changing and potentially damaging to our health and wellbeing. Each crisis, or *life change unit* (LCU), was given a different 'weighting' for stress based on its impact on our health. The more stressful life events we experience, the higher the cumulative score. The higher the score, the more likely we are to become ill.

The scores are cumulative, which helps us to understand why the death of a spouse is so stressful as the experience of loss may be compounded by other associated stressors (for example, the death of a spouse might add to our financial worries and changes to living conditions and our personal habits). In Table 8.2, we show the cumulative impact of stress for a person who has lost their partner and the additional impact that this may have on their financial, social and interpersonal worlds.

Life events stressors	LCU value
Death of a spouse	100
Change in financial state	38
Change in living conditions	25
Revision of personal habits	24
Revision of social activities	18
Change in eating habits	15

Table 8.2 An example of the cumulative effect of life events stress

LCU, life change unit.

This, according to Holmes and Rahe (1967), reveals an LCU stress score (220), which suggests a moderate to high chance of becoming ill in the near future.

Activity 8.2   Reflection

Life event stresses are rare but very impactful on our health and wellbeing. Think about a life event stress that you have experienced. What and who helped you to overcome these stresses? Why do you think this was helpful? How might this impact on your role as a nurse?

As this activity is based on your own reflection, no outline answer is provided at the end of the chapter.

Our personal vulnerability to stress

Our reactions to stress are highly personal and vary between people, so that exposure to the same event can provoke different reactions and can vary amongst people. Reactions to stress may differ *within* a person over time. That is, we may all have different responses to the same stressor at different times in our lives.

Our reactions to stress are not only based on our exposure to the different types of stressors discussed previously (*background stress* and *life event stress*), but are also dependent on our *personal vulnerability* to stress. This vulnerability arises from our personal history and previous experiences, which may predispose us to respond in a particular way in the face of a stressor. Our vulnerability, then, can vary depending on our:

- family and hereditary background;
- previous experience of coping with prior stressors;
- formative life experiences and exposure to role models;
- learned coping skills;
- attitudes, beliefs about our self, confidence, perceptions of our abilities;
- personality and temperament.

Our personality refers to a set of psychological characteristics which are relatively stable and which we use to define 'who we are'. Psychologists believe that if we have enough particular characteristics then this may describe our *personality type*. Our personality is shaped by genetic factors, early formative experiences (such as family dynamics), social influences and personal experiences. While these may be generally stable, it does not mean that aspects of our personality which are contributing to our problems are not amenable to change.

Some characteristics of our personality may make us more *prone* to stress:

- *type A personality characteristics* (aggressive, competitive, hostile, time-pressured);
- *co-dependent personality characteristics* (approval-seeking behaviour, perfectionist, martyr, feelings of inadequacy, reactionary);
- *helpless-hopeless personality characteristics* (external locus of control, compromised sense of agency, poor self-motivation, emotional dysregulation, negative thinking).

Some aspects of our personality make us more *resistant* to stress.

- *hardy personality characteristics* (solution-focused, takes control, sees opportunities rather than challenges) (Maddi and Kobasa, 1984);
- *survivor personality characteristics* (responds rather than reacts, optimist, creative problem-solving);
- *type 'R' personality characteristics* (taking calculated risks, adventurous spirit, sensation seeker) (Zuckerman, 2009).

Positive personal self-esteem (that is, a favourable, but realistic, view of our abilities and positive self-regard) also seems to protect us against stress, with some arguing that it is a psychological immune system (Branden, 1994).

Activity 8.3   Reflection

Resistance to stress

How resistant do you feel you are to stress? Make some notes about your personal characteristics which suggest to you that you are resilient to stress. Could this be improved? If so, how might you boost your personal resilience?

As this activity is based on your own reflection, no outline answer is provided at the end of the chapter.

What are the effects of stress?

Our response to stressors depends on our personal resources for coping and our resilience in stressful situations. While our bodies are well adapted to short periods of acute stress, prolonged distress causes cumulative wear and tear on our bodies (known as the *allostatic load*).

The effects of stress involve:

* *physical effects*: what our body does in response to stress;
* *emotional effects*: how we feel in response to stress;
* *psychological effects*: how we think about stress;
* *social and behavioural effects*: what we do in response to stress, how we cope.

Let's look at these in more depth.

Physical effects

Understanding the mechanisms which underpin our body's normal response to threat or fear can help us to understand and feel empowered to respond to our stress. Our *autonomic nervous system* is involuntary (that is, automatic) and conducts signals from our brain and spinal cord to our muscles, organs and glands. It comprises:

* *sympathetic nervous system* (which triggers fight or flight in response to threat);
* *parasympathetic nervous system* (which calms the body via release of hormones to return the body to balance).

Sympathetic activity is what we would recognise as 'stress', e.g. increased blood pressure, breathing and heart rate. This is normal and adaptive. If the sympathetic response persists and is repeatedly activated when we perceive an ongoing threat, we are experiencing *chronic* stress. This increases the risk for developing or exacerbating diseases such as diabetes, cancer, cardiovascular disease and hypertension.

There are a number of significant physical effects caused by the arousal of the sympathetic system, such as sleep disturbances, sweating and frequent urination. We may experience agitation, muscle tension, head, shoulder, back, dental or jaw problems (caused by grinding our teeth, known as *bruxism*), aches and pains. There may be gastrointestinal issues such as diarrhoea or constipation, stomach pains, bleeding, ulceration of stomach/colon (colitis), and irritable bowel syndrome (IBS) is known to be exacerbated, or even triggered, by stress.

Prolonged stress can also lead to nausea, dizziness, blurred vision, migraines and headaches, a loss of sex drive, chest pain, palpitations and elevated blood pressure, resulting in hypertension (high blood pressure) and atherosclerosis (narrowing and hardening of the arteries), both precursors to cardiovascular (heart) disease. The mechanisms for this are not completely clear but it seems that stress provokes an inflammatory response in the body which is associated with an increase in cytokines (chemical messengers secreted by our immune systems). Interleukin-6 (IL-6), for example, is a cytokine released in chronic stress which has been found to have a role in cardiovascular disease, increasing the risk for heart attacks, particularly for those who are younger and those with iron deficiency (Markousis-Mavrogenis et al., 2019).

Stress can also impact our immune systems. *Cortisol* is a hormone released at times of stress. It heightens our memory and attention; decreases our sensitivity to pain; increases blood sugar and blood pressure. However, long-term persistent stress increases cortisol levels, causing atrophy of the lymphatic glands (thymus, spleen, lymph nodes), thereby reducing our white blood cells. This compromises our ability to fight disease, leaving the body open to infection (such as respiratory diseases, coughs and colds).

Stress also impacts our brain in a number of ways. Cortisol decreases *serotonin* in the brain (the so-called 'happiness hormone'), affecting our feelings of wellbeing. The hippocampus is the part of the brain responsible for memory and learning and it appears to be damaged by repeated exposure to stress, decreasing memory and learning (cognitive failures). Stress in middle-aged women has been linked to the development of dementia (Alzheimer's disease) in later life (Johannson et al., 2010).

Emotional effects

As mentioned previously, stress can affect our mental wellbeing. We may feel low in mood, isolated, and experience fatigue and low energy levels. We may feel overwhelmed, with racing thoughts and constant worrying and experience agitation and an inability to relax. Often people report feeling angry and irritable, losing their temper frequently and having a short fuse.

Psychological effects

Stress can also have an effect on our thinking, concentration and ability to solve problems. People experiencing stress often report memory problems, absent-mindedness, slips of attention, distractibility and forgetfulness. These are known as *cognitive failures* (Broadbent et al., 1982). It is also not uncommon for people to experience a 'mental fog' where the ability to organise one's thoughts and problem-solving may be compromised (this is known as *cognitive disorganisation*).

Social and behavioural effects

People who feel stressed often report disruptions to their daily living activities, such as eating more or less, sleeping too much or too little and exercising less often. They may avoid or neglect their responsibilities and there may be an increase in nervous habits, such as nail biting or pacing. People may tend to isolate themselves more and avoid social contacts. Sometimes, alcohol, cigarettes or drugs may be used in an attempt to cope with stress and to relax, which ultimately adds to the stress load that we may bear, for reasons we shall see later.

Activity 8.4   Reflection

Effects of stress

When you experience stress, what effects does it have on you? Do you recognise any of the above effects in your own experience? How might you recognise these effects in others? How might this affect your work as a nurse?

As this activity is based on your own reflection, no outline answer is provided at the end of the chapter.

Key points to remember about stress

- Stress is not always negative – it can be helpful. Acute stress helps us to 'fight' or prepares us for 'flight'.
- Stress can be a problem when it becomes prolonged, chronic or following exposure to traumatic events.
- Our body tries to restore a calming balance once we feel the threat is over. If we feel the threat to us is not over, our body remains in a heightened state of readiness.
- Background stresses are daily hassles – those irritating, frustrating, distressing demands or practical difficulties which contribute to our overall stress levels.
- Life event stressors are rare but significantly distressing events in our lives, over which we have little control.
- Stress can have physical, emotional, psychological, social and behavioural effects on us.

Managing stress

There are many ways in which we can manage our stress, including various techniques as well as lifestyle. We will now explore these in more detail.

Stress management techniques

There are, of course, a number of therapeutic techniques to support relaxation and these can be helpful for managing stress as and when it arises. For example:

- guided visual imagery (involving visualising a pleasant, peaceful and relaxing scene such as a warm beach);
- progressive muscle relaxation (where muscles in the body are tensed and relaxed in turn – also known as Jacobson's relaxation technique);

- focused and controlled breathing (where we learn to take control of our breathing and to breathe from our diaphragm);
- yoga;
- meditation.

There are also some therapeutic approaches used in mental health care which may be helpful for managing stress such as:

- mindfulness-based stress reduction (MBSR) (originating in the 1970 work of Jon Kabat-Zinn, today MBSR uses meditation and mindful exercises as a means of awareness of self);
- autogenic therapy (involves using a set of mental exercises to concentrate passively on parts of your body to turn off the flight, fright or freeze response to stress and to restore a homeostatic balance within the body and mind).

Maintaining a good work–life balance

A work–life balance refers to the maintenance of balance between work responsibilities, home responsibilities and leisure time to achieve optimum happiness, health and wellbeing. When this balance is not maintained, individuals may experience increased stress, emotional exhaustion and burnout. The recent UK *Working Lives* survey from CIPD (2019) identified work–life balance as a pertinent problem affecting the UK workforce, with respondents admitting that their work often disrupted their family life. A quarter of individuals reported feeling unable to switch off during their downtime as they were thinking about work. Sometimes referred to as work–life integration, this balance between work responsibilities and home or family life is said to be approaching tipping point in many health professionals.

Research summary

A survey of 10,627 health care workers in the USA (Schwartz et al., 2019) explored work–life integration using a scale that measured work–life climate. The scale asks the following questions to establish how an individual's work may be affecting their work–life balance:

'During the past week, how often did this occur?'

- skipped a meal;
- ate a poorly balanced meal;
- worked through a day/shift without any breaks;
- arrived home late from work;
- had difficulty sleeping;
- slept less than 5 hours in a night;
- changed personal/family plans because of work;
- felt frustrated by technology.

Work–life climate varied by role, work setting, shift pattern and shift length. When comparing individuals from the top and bottom quartiles for work–life climate, good work–life integration was associated with better teamwork, better safety measures at work and lower personal burnout.

Although organisational factors predicted work–life culture, work–life integration was also dependent on an individual's ability to maintain separation between personal life and work. As mental health professionals, the stresses and emotional labour of work can easily spill into our home lives. But, according to the results, if an individual reported breaching the boundary of one work–life climate item they were likely to struggle to maintain boundaries in the other items too. Leaving all your stress at work can seem unrealistic; however, these results highlight the importance of making efforts to stay in control of these work–life boundaries.

As highlighted in the research summary above, self-awareness is key to maintaining balance. Frequently re-evaluating the demands of your job and home life and knowing where to direct your energy help you to maintain balance between home and work. Also, knowing your own goals, needs and rewards in terms of leisure time is important to maintaining balance and wellbeing. Leisure time is different to just using distractions to unwind such as watching television; it is partaking in activities that we find engaging, challenging, meaningful and enjoyable. However, finding the time and space to fully engage in leisure time is difficult, and a skill that we should all work on. Csikszentmihalyi (1990) describes the *autotelic* personality type: individuals who find it easier to 'live in the moment' and experience *flow*. *Flow* refers to the sense of being totally absorbed and focused on an activity, without distractions, to the point where you lose track of time. You may be able to think of times when you have experienced *flow* before. *Autotelic* individuals are said to be goal-directed, derive more pleasure from their leisure time and experience better wellbeing.

To become more *autotelic* Buettner et al. (2011) suggest practising the following:

- *Set challenging yet attainable goals* that match your interest and skill level, such as slowly increasing the time, intensity or incline of your bike ride, for example.
- *Learn to become immersed in an activity* by removing distractions. For example, choose to forgo listening to your music or podcast when riding your bike to focus on enjoying the activity.
- *Be in the moment* by practising being mindful and aware of your surroundings, observing the view of the forest, enjoying the sounds of the birds singing or noticing the smell of freshly cut grass while on your bike ride.

Maintaining your physical health and healthy lifestyle

Working in increasingly complex and demanding environments, physical wellbeing is crucial to the mental health of all nurses, contributing positively to the care of their patients. Good physical health, including a healthy diet, sufficient sleep and physical activity, contributes to an overall sense of balance. Mental health professionals should be aware of the possible effects their work may have on their own physical health and take action to negate these by avoiding unhelpful coping strategies (see section on helpful coping, below) and engaging in self-care. Self-care is not selfish or self-indulgent; it should be considered as an integral part of maintaining your wellbeing and balance. Engaging in self-care includes physical necessities such as maintaining good hygiene, diet and nutrition, being physically active and seeking medical care when needed. The term also encompasses emotional and spiritual self-care activities, which include anything you may find relaxing or calming like mindfulness or meditation. Self-care may be different for everyone but investing time in the activities that work for you is said to increase self-esteem, improve your immune system and reduce stress, contributing to better mental and physical health.

Research summary

As well as impacting work–life balance, irregular shift patterns can negatively impact sleep, leading to fatigue, reduced alertness and impaired physical wellbeing. Research has suggested that long-term shift work can contribute to adverse health outcomes, such as mental health issues, gastrointestinal problems and reduced cardiovascular health. Burch et al. (2009) explored the effects of shift work on health care workers, finding that night shift or irregular shift workers were more likely to experience sleep and gastrointestinal problems, take non-prescription medication and have poorer fitness in comparison to day workers.

However, it is unclear whether these health consequences were mostly due to unhealthy behaviours, lack of self-care or unhelpful coping strategies, like self-medicating with alcohol, rather than the shift work itself. The authors comment that there are modifiable behaviours and healthy ways of coping that may negate these negative consequences on our physical health. For instance, it is well documented that engaging in exercise has a beneficial effect on sleep.

Uncertainty and stress

We all encounter unexpected events in our working lives – this includes not only changes to our working environments but also the health of people that we care for. Frequent uncertainty about why things happen is known as *causal uncertainty* (Weary and Edwards, 1996). Individuals with high *causal uncertainty* feel unable to understand and predict what happens to them. These feelings stem from a lack of perceived control over life and tend to elicit the desire to regain control. However, if the attempts to reduce uncertainty are unsuccessful, this can cause negative emotions and learned helplessness. Chronic *causal uncertainty* has negative psychological impacts, such as depression and anxiety (Weary et al., 2001). Studies indicate that clinical placements are characterised by uncertainty. However, social support from other nursing staff and supervisors buffers the effects of uncertainty and role ambiguity on student nurses' satisfaction and protects their wellbeing (Galletta et al., 2017). The moderating role of colleague support is further discussed in the section on helpful coping, below.

Accommodation is a cognitive mechanism that allows us to escape from uncertainty by the adjustment of our goals by those issues which constrain us. *Accommodation* allows people to maintain high life satisfaction despite the number of stressors they face and limits the negative psychological effects of setbacks. We get better at this as we age, and *accommodation* is more difficult if a goal is central to your life or sense of identity (Brandtstädter and Rothermund, 2002). In reaction to a setback, an individual may accept their limited control over life events and adjust their goals accordingly; for instance, accepting the limitations of their knowledge of the situation and becoming resigned to the fact that they will not always know why things happen to them, adjusting their goals whilst taking comfort that they may believe that everything happens for a reason. Even when experiencing *causal uncertainty*, those who are high in accommodation disengage from their lack of control over an event and the need to identify the cause as they accept what has happened to them, adjusting themselves and their goals accordingly.

Brandtstädter and Rothermund (2002) believe that balance is key to achieving a 'good life', referring to the equilibrium between *accommodation* and *assimilation*. *Assimilation* describes the efforts and activities you employ to try to reach your life goals. *Accommodation*, as explained, is the act of adjusting our goals to life events. Having a goal is crucial to our wellbeing, providing motivation and giving structure to our lives, as we discuss more in the next section on personal, meaningful goals. However, goals can be sources of dissatisfaction if we fall short of our own expectations, and the goals cannot be reached. To maintain balance and life satisfaction, we must stay focused on our goals and remain driven to achieve them; however we must be flexible enough to change our plans in reaction to situations or events that are outside our control. This has been called the *stability–flexibility* dilemma.

In the case study below Imogen is struggling with many unknowns in her life; acceptance of her life situation could help her to deal with the disappointment of not achieving her goal of an anticipated degree classification.

Case study: Imogen

Imogen read the brief for one of her final assignments, knowing she needed a score over 70% to achieve the First grade she'd been hoping to achieve in her course. However, in the weeks prior to submission, Imogen separated from her partner very suddenly. She was going through a tough time emotionally; this was exacerbated by having to find somewhere

(Continued)

(Continued)

else to live. She managed to submit her assignment on time despite this; however, when she received her feedback, she had achieved 60%.

Knowing that a First-class degree was out of her reach, this setback felt like defeat and she wanted to give up. However, she took comfort in the fact that she had tried her best and submitted the completed assignment on time despite what was happening in her personal life and the practical challenges she was having to overcome. She accepted that the goal of achieving a First was now not possible, so she adjusted her goal accordingly. Knowing that she did not need the higher grade to secure a job opportunity after university, she carried on working towards achieving a Second-class degree.

Personal, meaningful goals

For many people, having clear and personally meaningful goals to aim for is an important part of their wellbeing. Without a sense of purpose, our lives can feel empty, and we may feel adrift. Our goals, whether they reflect our personal or working life, help us to define a sense of direction, purpose and meaning in our lives and a sense of accomplishment when we have reached them. Our goals must, however, be realistic and achievable, or we may feel a failure if we set them too high and they are out of our reach. Having goals which are realistic and personally meaningful helps us to develop a sense of mastery and control over our lives and to feel motivated by our efforts towards achieving our goals.

Activity 8.5   Reflection

Take some time to reflect upon the following points:

- How in control of your life do you feel? How might this undermine or promote your mental health?
- What are your goals for your life? Do you feel able to achieve them?
- How might you feel if you had no aim or purpose in your life? Or if you were unable to achieve those personal goals that you have set for yourself?

As this activity is based on your own reflection, no outline answer is provided at the end of the chapter.

Service user voice

All of the interactions that [mental health service users] have with professionals should be geared towards aiding their recovery as they have great needs and need positive role models who will not only help them but will act as guides. I myself have therapeutic relationships with a number of people in the hospital where I am a patient. For example, my psychologist, whom I see once a week, is very supportive of me. He always seems to understand me and has good insight into the type of person that I am and what motivates me. I also have an occupational therapist who is very efficient in getting me involved with work and study placements in the community and I have a good relationship with my named nurse too. She always takes the time to talk to me every week prior to ward round to ask me how I feel about things that have gone on during the week and what I hope will happen in the coming week. They are all very supportive of me and this really helps me a lot.

Helpful coping

Coping is a biological function of an organism that helps to deal with challenges and threats to avoid harm. However, people can respond to threats in adaptive (helpful) or maladaptive (unhelpful) ways, either reducing or amplifying the effects of stressful life events. Professor Ellen Skinner, an expert in coping and developmental psychology, proposes that the development of coping is based on many factors, including individual attributes such as temperament and reactions to stress coupled with social contexts (Skinner and Zimmer-Gembeck, 2016). Adverse life events and lived experiences contribute to the way we deal with difficult experiences; coping is an iterative process that grows and develops throughout our lifespan. There are also developmental shifts in ways of coping; for example, children from the age of 4 increasingly seek support from peers rather than their caregivers.

Helpful coping supports our personal resilience, defined as the *ability to bounce back or positively adapt in the face of significant adversity or risk* (Snyder et al., 2011, page 114). Of course, the issue here is to consider, what people are actually 'bouncing back' to? There is a danger of specifying what may be considered within the normal range of human functioning and we should consider that any measure of resilience considers the individual and cultural context of individuals (Snyder et al., 2011). For Friedli (2009), there are three broad dimensions that support resilience and confer protection in times of adversity:

1. *environmental resources*: features of the natural and built environment that support communal capacity for resilience;
2. *social resources*: social networks and family life that enhance resilience amongst people and communities (see below);
3. *personal emotional and cognitive resources* that support and contribute to developing resilience amongst individuals, such as good mental health (factors which undermine personal resilience include mental distress, low levels of mental wellbeing and neglect of self and others and a range of unhelpful coping mechanisms and self-harming behaviours, including self-sedation and, for example, self-medication through alcohol and drugs, high fat and sugar consumption).

As suggested by the above definitions, our personal sense of mental wellbeing is also likely to be associated with our positive interpersonal relationships and environmental contexts. For many people, positive interpersonal relationships are assets that *protect* them from psychological harm and distress, *promote* their mental wellbeing and satisfaction with life and *support* resilience at times of adversity. This is likely to involve our ability to establish and maintain positive, warm, close, supportive and trusting interpersonal relationships. For Ryff (1989) and Ryff and Keyes (1995), this also includes an ability to compromise, a sense of empathy and compassion for others and an understanding of the ebb and flow of human relationships. Danzinger (1976) identified a classification of positive relationships based on:

* *solidarity* (a sense of belonging and interpersonal integration, social acceptance within a community and a common commitment between people and sharing resources);
* *intimacy* (people relating to one another as sources of personal satisfaction, including kindness, altruism, love, empathy, attachment);
* *influence* (recognising the relevance of social status and standing within a community or group).

In the case study below, Christine is affected by social and interpersonal aspects of her current life situation; widening her social circle may have positive benefits for her mental health and wellbeing.

Case study: Christine

Christine is a first-year nursing student in her late 50s and was widowed last year. She has recently enrolled on the BSc(Hons) adult nursing programme at her local university, realising her life's ambition to become a nurse. One of her adult children has emigrated to Australia and has a young family there. The other lives in London, over 100 miles away, and works very long hours in a high-pressure city job. For the last 2 years of her husband's life, Christine was his carer and she put her aspiration to become a nurse on hold to care for him. She dropped out of her usual social activities such as the art club and book group. Now she feels very isolated and has become depressed.

Marta, a friend of hers on the course, sees that Christine is often sad and tearful. She decides to try and talk to Christine about what is troubling her. At Christine's house, Marta asks about a painting hanging on the living-room wall. Christine mentions that she painted it herself and used to enjoy her art, but she has lost the knack now, and has lost touch with her friends from the group. Marta encourages Christine to make contact again with some of them, and in return Christine invites Marta to come along with her, which she accepts, recognising that she too could benefit from widening her social circle.

Certain ways of coping, such as problem-solving, negotiation and focusing on the positives, are 'adaptive', decreasing psychological distress and promoting physical and mental health and wellbeing. Other ways of dealing with stress, including avoidance, rumination or venting, are viewed as 'maladaptive'; associated with mental disorder and distress. However, the families cannot necessarily all be clearly divided into 'adaptive' or 'maladaptive' strategies. For instance, help-seeking and support-seeking can have inconsistent outcomes, depending on the helpfulness of the advice given. As the families of coping suggest, individuals draw both upon their own resources and social resources (such as support from others) for coping. With the notion that your coping mechanisms can exacerbate your problems, it is important to focus on improving your own coping, not just solving any issue you are currently facing. This means that you are learning ways to better equip yourself to solve future problems.

Research summary

Labrague et al. (2018) conducted a systematic review of 13 studies researching coping strategies in nursing students. Stress levels in the nursing students from all years of study ranged from moderate to high. Main stressors identified included stress through the caring of patients, assignments, workloads and negative social interactions with staff and faculty. Of the studies included, six found that problem-solving was the main approach in dealing with stress. This family of coping is considered the most effective way of dealing with stress, involving planning, setting objectives and using past experiences to solve a problem. Other studies reported talking to relatives and friends was a frequently used way of coping. However, many studies reported that the nursing students used transference such as exercise, watching TV and eating. These strategies to deal with stress were ineffective as they do not address the cause of stress. Other studies found that nursing students tended to opt for maladaptive ways of coping during times of stress, such as ignoring their stress or separating themselves from others. The stress experienced by nursing students can have detrimental effects on nurses and their patients so it is important to consider the ways in which we cope with stress.

Schreuder et al. (2012) investigated coping styles of nurses. Active coping, such as problem-solving, had a positive correlation with general health, mental health, job control and job support. High scores on passive coping (avoiding problems or waiting to see what happens) correlated with poor general health, poor mental health, high job demands, low job control and low job support. Passive coping was found to relate to poor general health, poor mental health, low job control and low job support. The nurses with passive coping styles tended to experience low social support. An important part of our coping as nurses is through the support of other nurses and the wider multiprofessional team. Support-seeking behaviours include contact which has an emotional, restorative function but also for help, information, guidance and advice (instrumental aid). Much of this support is informal in nursing – the formalised version of such support is clinical supervision. Unfortunately, while there is a considerable body of evidence that indicates how clinical supervision may support nurses' wellbeing and resilience, combating burnout and stress, there is also sadly evidence that it remains underutilised amongst nursing teams (Markey et al., 2020).

More effective ways of coping can be learned through interventions that target problem-solving, emotional regulation, cognitive restructuring or mindfulness. Research suggests that these types of interventions can significantly improve psychological outcomes. In a randomised controlled trial, undergraduate students participated in resilience and coping sessions where they were encouraged to explore their thoughts and feelings relating to their problems, brainstorm options for change and develop action plans. After this 3-week intervention students reported significantly more hope and less stress and depression in comparison to the control group (Houston et al., 2017). Additionally, 93% of participants felt that they could now make helpful choices when faced with problems (First et al., 2018).

Activity 8.6 Developing your stress toolkit

Bearing in mind the above information, consider your coping styles.

- How would you build on your positive, adaptive helpful coping styles?
- How might you seek to enhance your resilience?
- How might clinical supervision help to reduce your stress and maintain your wellbeing?

As this activity is based on your own reflection, no outline answer is provided at the end of the chapter.

Our positive wellbeing

If we feel that we have positive mental wellbeing we may have a sense of our own personal autonomy in that we feel we have control of and manage our lives and have a sense of being able to rely on ourselves to cope in times of trouble. The experience of being in control of our own lives is one which most adults enjoy and take for granted. There may also be an acceptance of ourselves and our life and our personal experiences, along with the highs and lows of life's events and our abilities as well as limitations (Ryff, 1989; Ryff and Keyes, 1995). The ability to take available opportunities and to enjoy a family life or to have a 'working life' which contributes to wider society, to be part of a local community and to have access to services which contribute to a person's sense of security and wellbeing, are all principles which most people hold dear.

The experience of mental ill health can have a profound effect on all of these aspects of our lives, even to the point of no longer feeling that we have any sense of control over our own life decisions and that our opinion is not only ignored, but worse, it is never sought in the first instance (Repper and Perkins, 2003). All experiences change us and reframe our world and the 'illness' experience is just the same. Conversely, the practice of discussing recovery, sharing the knowledge that it is personally defined, acknowledging that people take varied routes and lengths of times and the journey contains setbacks and difficulties but that it is to be expected and supported, is therapeutic and inspiring.

Activity 8.7   Reflection on your skills and talents

List your skills, abilities and talents. What do you think you are best at? How does this contribute to your happiness and satisfaction with life? How many of these benefit your practice as a nurse?

Now, take some time to consider what your vulnerabilities to stress might be. Consider your genetic/family background and life experiences.

As this activity is based on your own reflection, no outline answer is provided at the end of the chapter.

What are strengths? For Park et al. (2004, page 603), our character strengths are *positive traits reflected in thoughts, feelings, and behaviours* which are associated with mental wellbeing. Strengths are the personal and social capital that supports our resilience and our ability to cope at times of uncertainty, protecting us from psychological harm, and thereby allowing us to flourish. An individual who is flourishing in this sense may be seen as someone who is thriving in their world. The person may feel that they are in charge of their life, with a sense of autonomy, and that they believe they have the personal and social resources and abilities to be resilient and cope with life's troubles. There might be a sense of personal accomplishment, environmental mastery and personal growth. A person may feel that their talents, knowledge and skills are strengths in that they provide opportunities for them to meet their aspirations or pursue their personal interests.

Attempting to identify an individual's strengths and abilities is a challenge as people often find it is easier (and quicker) to describe their perceived weaknesses (Snyder et al., 2011). This is also a challenge perhaps for mental health practitioners who are most used to assessing psychological deficits (Peterson and Seligman, 2004).

A number of tools have attempted to assist people to identify their strengths. For example, the self-report questionnaire Clifton Strengths Finder (Buckingham and Clifton, 2001) (available for purchase at www.strengthsfinder.com) identifies 34 strength themes such as communication (the ability to put one's thoughts into action), restorative (being able to resolve challenges) and analytical (understanding reasons and causes).

Other self-report questionnaires include the Values in Action (VIA) Brief Strengths Test (24 questions which take approximately 5 minutes to complete) and the longer VIA Survey of Character Strengths (taking approximately 15 minutes) (Peterson and Seligman, 2004) (both available free of charge after registration at: www.viacharacter.org/), such as bravery, citizenship, creativity, fairness and integrity. These surveys reveal an individual's personal strengths. This helps people to understand their characters better and subsequently to take advantage of their positive personal qualities in enhancing their everyday lives (Snyder et al., 2011).

Activity 8.8   Reflection on your character strengths

Register for, and take, the VIA Character Strengths test (www.viacharacter.org/).

How many of the strengths outlined in the VIA Survey do you feel you have? How many would you like to develop?

As this activity is based on your own reflection, no outline answer is provided at the end of the chapter.

Chapter summary

In this chapter we have considered your mental health and wellbeing as an adult nurse and, in particular, the ways in which you can maintain your wellbeing. We have explored the different types of stress we may experience and the pervasive impact of stress on our personal and working lives. We have looked at adaptive and maladaptive coping and how we can develop our own stress management toolkit. The issue of personal resilience, which features in the new nursing curricula, has been discussed along with how nursing students can promote their own positive wellbeing by adopting a mentally healthy lifestyle.

Further reading

Van der Kolk, B (2014) *The Body Keeps the Score*. London: Penguin.

This book explores how trauma and stress can have a significant and lasting impact on our minds and bodies and the paths to recovery that we can take to help let go of painful memories and experiences.

References

American Psychiatric Association (APA) (2013) *Diagnostic and Statistical Manual of Mental Disorders* (5th ed.). Available online at: https://doi.org/10.1176/appi.books.9780890425596 (accessed 19 January 2022).

Anderson, IM, Ferrier, IN, Baldwin, RC, Cowen, PJ, Howard, L, Lewis G, Matthews, K, McAllister-Williams, RH, Peveler, RC, Scott, J and Tyler, A (2008) Evidence-based guidelines for treating depressive disorders with antidepressants: A revision of the 2000 British Association for Psychopharmacology guidelines. *Journal of Psychopharmacology*, 22 (4): 343–96.

Attoe, C, Lillywhite, K, Hinchliffe, E, Bazley, A and Cross, S (2018) Integrating mental and physical health care: The mind and body approach. *The Lancet Psychiatry*, 5 (5): 387–9. https://doi.org/10.1016/S2215-0366(18)30044-0

Ball, JS, Links, PS, Strike, C and Boydell, KM (2005) 'It's overwhelming … everything seems to be too much': A theory of crisis for individuals with severe persistent mental illness. *Psychiatric Rehabilitation Journal*, 29 (1): 10–17.

Barker, P and Barker-Buchanan, P (2011) Myth of mental health nursing and the challenge of recovery. *International Journal of Mental Health Nursing*, 20: 337–44.

Barnes RD, Ivezaj V, Martino S, Pitman, BP, Paris, M and Grilo, CM (2021) 12 Months later: Motivational interviewing plus nutrition psychoeducation for weight loss in primary care. *Eating and Weight Disorders: EWD*, 26 (6): 2077–81. https://doi.org/10.1007/s40519-020-00994-5

Barnett, P, Mackay, E, Matthews, H, Gate, R, Greenwood, H, Ariyo, K, Bhui, K, Halvorsrud, K, Pilling, S and Smith, S (2019) Ethnic variations in compulsory detention under the Mental Health Act: A systematic review and meta-analysis of international data, *Lancet Psychiatry*, 6: 305–17. http://dx.doi.org/10.1016/S2215-0366(19)30027-6

Beck, A (1976) *Cognitive Therapy and the Emotional Disorders*. New York: International University Press.

Bennaman, L (2012) Crisis emergencies for individuals with severe, persistent mental illnesses: A situation-specific theory. *Archives of Psychiatric Nursing*, 26 (4): 251–260.

Benner, P (1984) *From Novice to Expert: Excellence and Power in Clinical Nursing Practice.* London: Addison Wesley.

Bentall, R (2003) *Madness Explained: Psychosis and Human Nature.* London: Penguin.

Berner, P, Bezner, JR, Morris, D and Lein, DH (2021) Nutrition in physical therapist practice: Tools and strategies to act now. *Physical Therapy*, 101 (5): 1–9.

Bonanno, GA and Mancini, AD (2008) The human capacity to thrive in the face of potential trauma. *Pediatrics*, 121 (2).

Borsari, B, Li, Y, Tighe, J, Manuel, JK, Gⓧkbayrak, NS, Delucchi, K, Moaraso, BJ, Abadjian, L, Cohen, BE, Baxley, C and Seal, KH (2021) A pilot trial of collaborative care with motivational interviewing to reduce opioid risk and improve chronic pain management. *Addiction*, 116 (9): 2387–97. https://doi.org/10.1111/add.15401

Branden, N (1994) *The Six Pillars of Self-Esteem.* New York: Random House.

Brandtstädter, J and Rothermund, K (2002) The life-course dynamics of goal pursuit and goal adjustment: A two-process framework. *Developmental Review*, 22 (1): 117–50.

Brannelly, T (2011) Sustaining citizenship: People with dementia and the phenomenon of social death. *Nursing Ethics*, 18 (5): 662–71.

Brannelly, T (2015) Mental health service use and the ethics of care: In pursuit of justice, in *Ethics of Care: Critical Advances in International Perspective* (pp. 219–32). Bristol: Policy Press.

Brannelly, T (2016) Citizenship and people living with dementia: A case for the ethics of care. *Dementia, The International Journal of Social Research and Practice*, 15 (3): 304–14.

Brannelly, T (2019) An ethics of care transformation of mental health service provision: Creating services that people want to use, in *Ethics from the Ground Up: Emerging Debates, Changing Practices and New Voices in Healthcare*. London: Red Globe Press.

Breland, JY, Hundt, NE, Barrera, TL, Mignogna, J, Petersen, NJ, Stanley, MA and Cully, JA (2015) Identification of anxiety symptom clusters in patients with COPD: Implications for assessment and treatment. *International Journal of Behavioural Medicine*, 22: 590–6.

Broadbent, DE, Cooper, PF, FibGerald, P and Parkes, K (1982) The Cognitive Failures Questionnaire (CFQ) and its correlates. *British Journal of Clinical Psychology*, 21: 1–16.

Brown, A (2006) Prenatal infection as a risk factor for schizophrenia. *Schizophrenia Bulletin*, 32 (2): 200–2.

Brown, G and Harris, T (1978) *The Social Origins of Depression: A Study of Psychiatric Disorder in Women.* London: Tavistock.

Buckingham, M and Clifton, DO (2001) *Now, Discover your Strengths: How to Develop Your Talents and Those of the People you Manage.* London: Simon & Schuster.

Buettner, L, Shattell, M and Reber, M (2011) Working hard to relax: Improving engagement in leisure time activities for a healthier work–life balance. *Issues in Mental Health Nursing*, 32 (4): 269–70.

Burch, JB, Tom, J, Zhai, Y, Criswell, L, Leo, E and Ogoussan, K (2009) Shiftwork impacts and adaptation among health care workers. *Occupational Medicine*, 59 (3): 159–66.

Burke Harris, N (2014) How childhood trauma affects health across a lifetime. TED talk.

Cameron, D, Kapur, R and Campbell, P (2005) Releasing the therapeutic potential of the psychiatric nurse: A human relations perspective of the nurse–patient relationship. *Journal of Psychiatric and Mental Health Nursing*, 12: 64–74.

Cancer Research UK (2021) *Cancer Risk Statistics.* Available online at: www.cancerresearchuk.org/health-professional/cancer-statistics/risk#heading-Two. (accessed 30 August 2021).

Caplan, G (1989) Recent developments in crisis intervention and the promotion of support service. *Journal of Primary Prevention*, 10 (1): 3–25.

Care Quality Commission (2015) *Right Here, Right Now: People's Experiences of Help, Care and Support During a Mental Health Crisis.* London: CQC.

Chelvanayagam, S and James, J (2018) What is diabulimia and what are the implications for practice? *British Journal of Nursing*, 27 (17): 980–6.

Chelvanayagam, S and Newell, C (2015) Differentiating between eating disorders and gastrointestinal problems. *Gastrointestinal Nursing* 13 (7): 56–62.

Chelvanayagam, S, Tuck, J and Eales, S (2020) Recognising anxiety and depression in patients with long-term physical conditions. *General Practice Nursing*, 6 (3): 60–8.

Chen, H-M, Lee, H-L, Yang, F-C, Chiu, Y-W and Chao, S-Y (2020) Effectiveness of motivational interviewing in regard to activities of daily living and motivation for rehabilitation among stroke patients. *International Journal of Environmental Research and Public Health*, 17 (8). doi:10.3390/ijerph17082755

CIPD (2019) *UK Working Lives: The CIPD Job Quality Index.* Available online at: www.cipd.co.uk/Images/uk-working-lives-summary-2019-v1_tcm18-58584.pdf (accessed 17 June 2021).

Cipriani, A, Smith, K, Burgess, S, Carney, S, Goodwin, G and Geddes, J (2006) Lithium versus antidepressants in the long-term treatment of unipolar affective disorder. *The Cochrane Database of Systematic Reviews*, 4: CD003492.

Clarke, M, Davies, S, Hollin, C and Duggan, C (2011) Long-term suicide risk in forensic psychiatric patients. *Archives of Suicide Research*, 15 (1): 16–28. DOI: 10.1080/13811118.2011.539951

Cohen, BE, Edmondson, D and Kronish, IM (2015) State of the art review: Depression, stress, anxiety, and cardiovascular disease. *American Journal of Hypertension*, 28 (11): 1295–302.

Cook, N, Shepherd, A and Boore, J (2021) *Essentials of Anatomy and Physiology for Nursing Practice* (2nd ed.). London: SAGE.

Craig, TJ (2008) Major psychiatric disorders increase risk of mortality. *Evidence Based Mental Health*, 11. DOI:10.1 136/ebrnh.11.1.9

Csikszentmihalyi, M (1990) *Flow: The Psychology of Optimal Experience.* New York: Harper Collins.

CSIP Acute Programme and Change Agent Team (2007) *A Positive Outlook: A Good Practice Toolkit to Improve Discharge from Inpatient Mental Health Care.* York: CSIP.

Cutcliffe, JR and Koehn, CV (2007) Hope and interpersonal psychiatric/mental health nursing: A systematic review of the literature – Part II. *Journal of Psychiatric and Mental Health Nursing*, 14: 141–7.

Danzinger, K (1976) *Interpersonal Communication.* Oxford: Pergamon Press.

Davies, SC (2015) *Annual Report of the Chief Medical Officer 2015. On the State of the Public's Health, Baby Boomers: Fit for the Future.* London: Department of Health.

Dayson, C and Bashir, N (2014) *The Social and Economic Impact of the Rotherham Social Prescribing Pilot Main Evaluation Report.* Sheffield: Sheffield Hallam University.

De Vries, J and Timmins, F (2017) *Understanding Psychology for Nursing Students.* London: SAGE.

Dennett, C (2021) What is the gut–brain reaction? Why having a "gut feeling" is more than just an expression. *Environmental Nutrition*, 44 (9): 4.

Department of Health (2004) *The Ten Essential Shared Capabilities: A Framework for the Whole of the Mental Health Workforce.* London: Department of Health.

Department of Health (2011) *No Health Without Mental Health – A Cross-Government Mental Health Outcomes Strategy for People of All Ages.* Available online at: www.gov.uk/government/publications/no-health-without-mental-health-a-cross-government-outcomes-strategy

Department of Health (2014) *Closing the Gap: Priorities for Essential Change in Mental Health.* Available online at: https://assets.publishing.service.gov.uk/government/uploads/system/uploads/attachment_data/file/281250/Closing_the_gap_V2_-_17_Feb_2014.pdf

Dew, K, Morgan, S, Dowell, A, McLeod, I, Bushnell, J and Collings, S (2007) It puts things out of your control: Fear of consequences as a barrier to patient disclosure of mental health issues to general practitioners. *Sociology of Health and Illness*, 29 (7): 1059–74. DOI: 1O.1111/j.1467-9566.2007.01022.x.

Donald, EE and Stajduhar, KI (2019) A scoping review of palliative care for persons with severe persistent mental illness. *Palliative and Supportive Care*, 1–9.

Doyle, EA, Quinn, SM, Ambrosino, JM, Weyman, K, Tamborlane, WV and Jastreboff, AM (2017) Disordered eating behaviors in emerging adults with type 1 diabetes: A common problem for both men and women. *Journal of Pediatric Health Care*, 31 (3): 327–33.

Durkheim, E. (1897) *Suicide: A Study in Sociology* (1951 edition, Spaulding, JA and Simpson, G, trans.). London: Routledge.

Dury, R (2015) Mental and physical long-term conditions in the UK: Spanning the boundaries. *British Journal of Community Nursing*, 20 (4): 190–3.

Elassal, G, Elsheikh, M, Gawad, A and Zeid, A (2013) Assessment of depression and anxiety symptoms in chronic obstructive pulmonary disease patients: A case–control study. *Egyptian Journal of Chest Diseases and Tuberculosis*, 63: 575–82.

Engel, G (1977) The need for a new medical model. *Science*, 196: 129–36.

Felitti, V (2002) The relation between adverse childhood experiences and adult health: Turning gold into lead. *The Permanente Journal*, 6 (1): 44–7.

Felton, A and Stacey, G (2008) Positive risk taking: A framework for practice, in Sickley, T and Basset, T (eds) *Learning About Mental Health Practice.* Chichester: Wiley.

First, J, First, NL and Houston, JB (2018) Resilience and coping intervention (RCI): A group intervention to foster college student resilience. *Social Work with Groups*, 41 (3): 198–210.

Fisher, D (2008) Promoting recovery. In Stickley, T and Basset, T (eds) *Learning About Mental Health Practice* (pp. 119–41). Chichester: Wiley.

Fond, G, Salas, S, Pauly, V, Baumstark, K, Bernard, C, Orleans, V, Llorca, P-M, Lancon, C, Auquier, P and Boyer, L (2019) End of life care among patients with schizophrenia and cancer: A population-based cohort study from the French national hospital database. *The Lancet*, 4L e583–91.

Fransella, F and Dalton, P (2000) *Personal Construct Counselling in Action* (2nd edition). London: SAGE.

Friedli, L (2009) *Mental Health, Resilience and Inequalities*. Denmark: World Health Organization Europe.

Future Vision Coalition (2009) *A Future Vision for Mental Health*. Available online at: www.mentalhealth.org.uk/policy/future-vision-coalition-new-mental-health-strategy (accessed 19 January 2022).

Gaglioti, AH, Barlow, P, DuChene Thoma, K and Bergus, GR (2017) Integrated care coordination by an interprofessional team reduces emergency department visits and hospitalisations at an academic health centre. *Journal of Interprofessional Care*, 31 (5): 557–65.

Gajwani, R, Parsons, H, Birchwood, M and Singh, SP (2016) Ethnicity and detention: Are Black and minority ethnic (BME) groups disproportionately detained under the Mental Health Act 2007? *Social Psychiatry and Psychiatric Epidemiology*, 51: 703–11. DOI: 10.1007/s00127-016-1118-z

Galletta, M, Portoghese, I, Gonzales, CIA, Melis, P, Marcias, G, Campagna, M ... and Sardu, C (2017) Lack of respect, role uncertainty and satisfaction with clinical practice among nursing students: The moderating role of supportive staff. *Acta Bio Medica: Atenei Parmensis*, 88 (Suppl 3): 43.

Gilligan, C (1982) *In a Different Voice: Psychological Theory and Women's Development*. Cambridge, MA: Harvard University Press.

Glover-Thomas, N (2011) The age of risk: Risk perception and determination following the Mental Health Act 2007. *Medical Law Review*, 19: 581–605.

Goldberg, H (1977) *The Hazards of Being Male: Surviving the Myth of Masculine Privilege*. New York: Signet Books.

Green. L (2010) *Understanding the Life Course: Sociological and Psychological Perspectives*. Cambridge: Polity Press.

Gross, R and Kinson, N (2007) *Psychology for Nurses and Allied Health Professionals*. Oxford: Hodder Arnold.

Harper, B, Dickson, JM and Bramwell, R (2014) Experiences of young people in a 16–18 Mental Health Service. *Child and Adolescent Mental Health*, 19 (2): 90–6.

Hassed, C (2004) Bringing holism into mainstream biomedical education. *Journal of Alternative and Complementary Medicine*, 10 (2): 405–7.

Heald, AH, Stedman, M, Davies, M, Livingston, M, Taylor, D and Gadsby, R (2020) Antidepressant prescribing in England: Patterns and costs. *Primary Care Companion for CNS Disorders*, 16: 22 (2).

Health and Safety Executive (HSE) (2019) *Tackling Work-Related Stress Using the Management Standards Approach.* Available online at: www.hse.gov.uk/pubns/wbk01.pdf

Her Majesty's Government/Department of Health (HMG/DH) (2011) *No Health Without Mental Health.* Available online at: www.gov.uk/government/uploads/system/uploads/attachment_data/file/213761/dh_124058.pdf

Hewitt, J and Coffey, M (2005) Therapeutic working relationships with people with schizophrenia: Literature review. *Journal of Advanced Nursing,* 52 (5): 561–70.

Higgins, A and McBennett, P (2007) The petals of recovery in a mental health context. *British Journal of Nursing,* 16 (14): 852–6.

Hill, N, Olalekan, K, Thyagarajan, R, Freeman, A, Coles, L and Waine, J (2018) *Rapid Tranquillisation and the Management of Violent and Aggressive Paediatric Patients.* London: PIER Network.

Holland, L (2018) *The Nurse's Guide to Mental Health Medicines.* London: SAGE.

Holmes, T and Rahe, R (1967) The social readjustment rating scale. *Journal of Psychosomatic Research,* 11 (2): 213–18.

Houston, JB, First, J, Spialek, ML, Sorenson, ME, Mills-Sandoval, T, Lockett, M, First, NL, Nitiéma, P, Allen, SF and Pfefferbaum, B (2017) Randomized controlled trial of the Resilience and Coping Intervention (RCI) with undergraduate university students. *Journal of American College Health,* 65 (1): 1–9.

Howard League for Penal Reform (2016) *Preventing Prison Suicide.* Available online at: https://howardleague.org/wp-content/uploads/2016/11/Preventing-prison-suicide-report.pdf

Illich, I (1975) *Medical Nemesis.* London: Calder & Boyars.

Iveson, C (2002) Solution-focused brief therapy. *Advances in Psychiatric Treatment,* 8: 149–56.

Jerwood, J, Phimister, D, Ward, G et al. (2018) Barriers to palliative care for people with severe mental illness: Exploring the views of clinical staff. *European Journal of Palliative Care,* 25 (1): 20–5.

Johannson, L, Guo, X, Waern, M, Ostling, S, Gustafson, D, Bengtsson, C and Skoog, I (2010) Midlife psychological stress and risk of dementia: A 35-year longitudinal population study. *Brain,* 133: 2217–24.

Johnson, S, Lamb, D, Marston, L, Osborn, D, Mason, O, Henderson, C et al. (2018) Peer-supported self-management for people discharged from a mental health crisis team: A randomised controlled trial. *The Lancet,* 392: 409–18.

Johnstone, L and Boyle, M (2018) *The Power Threat Meaning Framework: Towards the Identification of Patterns in Emotional Distress, Unusual Experiences and Troubled or Troubling Behaviour, as an Alternative to Functional Psychiatric Diagnosis.* Leicester: British Psychological Society.

Joint Formulary Committee (2021) *British National Formulary* (81st edition). London: BMJ Group and Pharmaceutical Press.

Jonas, W and Rosenbaum, E (2021) The case for whole-person integrative care. *Medicina*, 57 (677): 677. DOI: 10.3390/Medicina57070677.

Judd, LL, Akiskal, HS, Schettler, PJ, Endicott, J, Maser, J, Solomon, DA, Leon, AC, Rice, JA and Keller, MB (2002) The long-term natural history of the weekly symptomatic status of bipolar I disorder. *Archives of General Psychiatry*, 59 (6): 530–7.

Judd, LL, Akiskal, HS, Schettler, PJ, Coryell, W, Endicott, J, Maser, JD, Solomon, DA, Leon, AC and Keller, MB (2003) A prospective investigation of the natural history of the long-term weekly symptomatic status of bipolar II disorder. *Archives of General Psychiatry*, 60 (3): 261–9.

Kanner, A, Coyne, JC, Schaefer, C and Lazarus, RS (1981) Comparison of two modes of stress measurement: Daily hassles and uplifts versus major life events. *Journal of Behavioral Medicine*, 4 (1): 1–39.

Kelly, G (1955/1991) *The Psychology of Personal Constructs. Volume 1: Theory and Personality*. London: Routledge.

Khan, M, Twigg, J and Chin, R (2021) A journey to compassion: A service-user perspective. *Clinical Psychology Forum*, 337: 63–7.

Konstantinou, P, Kassianos, AP, Georgiou, G, Panayides, A, Papageorgiou, A, Almas, I, Wozniak, G and Karekla, M (2020) Barriers, facilitators, and interventions for medication adherence across chronic conditions with the highest non-adherence rates: A scoping review with recommendations for intervention development. *Translational Behavioral Medicine*, 10 (6): 1390–8. DOI: 10.1093/tbm/ibaa118.

Kring, A and Johnson, S (2019) *Abnormal Psychology: The Science and Treatment of Psychological Disorders* (14th edition). Hoboken, NJ: Wiley.

Kunitz, S (2002) Holism and the idea of general susceptibility to disease. *International Journal of Epidemiology*, 31: 722–9.

Labrague, LJ, McEnroe-Petitte, DM, Al Amri, M, Fronda, DC and Obeidat, AA (2018) An integrative review on coping skills in nursing students: Implications for policymaking. *International Nursing Review*, 65: 279–291.

Lazarus, RS (1999) *Stress and Emotion: A New Synthesis*. New York: Springer.

Leibman, RE and Burnette, M (2013) It's not you, it's me: An examination of clinician- and client-level influences on countertransference toward borderline personality disorder. *American Journal of Orthopsychiatry*, 83 (1): 115–25.

Leventhal, H, Benyamini, Y, Brownlee, S, Diefenbach, M and Leventhal, EA (1997) Illness representations: Theoretical foundations, perceptions of health and illness, in Petrie, KJ, Weinman, JA (eds) *Perceptions of Health and Illness: Current Research and Applications* (pp. 19–46). Amsterdam: Harwood Academic.

Lindström, B and Eriksson, M (2005) Salutogenesis. *Journal of Epidemiology and Community Health*, 59: 440–2.

Littrell, J (2008) The mind–body connection: Not just a theory any more. *Social Work in Health Care*, 46 (4).

Lovelock, J (2001) *Homage to Gaia: The Life of an Independent Scientist.* Oxford: Oxford University Press.

Maddi, SR and Kobasa, SC (1984) *The Hardy Executive: Health Under Stress.* Homewood, IL: Dow Jones-Irwin.

Majed, B, Arveiler, D, Bingham, A, et al. (2012) Depressive symptoms: A time-dependent risk factor for coronary heart disease and stroke in middle-aged men. The PRIME study. *Stroke*, 43: 1761–7.

Mancini, M (2007) The role of self-efficacy in recovery from serious psychiatric disabilities. *Qualitative Social Work*, 6 (1): 49–74.

Margereson, C and Trenoweth, S (2010) Epidemiology and aetiology of long-term conditions, in Margereson, C and Trenoweth, S (eds) *Developing Holistic Care for Long-Term Conditions.* London: Routledge.

Markey, K, Murphy, L, O'Donnell, C, Turner, J and Doody, O (2020) Clinical supervision: A panacea for missed care. *Journal of Nursing Management*, 28: 2113–17.

Markousis-Mavrogenis, G, Tromp, J, Ouwerkerk, W, Devalaraja, M, Anker, SD, Cleland, JG et al. (2019) The clinical significance of interleukin-6 in heart failure: Results from the BIOSTAT-CHF study. *European Journal of Heart Failure*, 21 (8): 965–73. DOI: 10.1002/ejhf.1482

Martin, P, Patel, V, Shekhar, S, Mario, M, Maselko, J and Rahman, A (2007) No health without mental health. *The Lancet*, 370 (9590): 859–77.

Maslakpak, MH, Parizad, N, Ghahremani, A and Alinejad, V (2021) The effect of motivational interviewing on the self-efficacy of people with type 2 diabetes: A randomised controlled trial. *Journal of Diabetes Nursing*, 25 (4): 1–8.

Maté, G (2019) *When the Body Says No: The Cost of Hidden Stress.* London: Penguin.

Matthews, J (2008) The meaning of recovery, in: Lynch, J and Trenoweth, S (eds) *Contemporary Issues in Mental Health Nursing.* Chichester: Wiley.

McAuliffe, D and Chenoweth, L (2008) Leave no stone unturned: The inclusive model of ethical decision making. *Ethics and Social Welfare*, 2 (1): 38–49. DOI: 10.1080/17496530801948739

McEwen, B and Fenasse, R (2019) Probiotics and depression: The link between the microbiome–gut–brain axis and digestive and mental health. *Journal of the Australian Traditional-Medicine Society*, 25 (3): 127–32.

Mehta, N (2011) Mind–body dualism: A critique from a health perspective. *Mens Sana Monographs*, 9 (1): 202–9.

Mental Health Foundation (2006) *Feeding Minds.* Available online at: www.mentalhealth.org.uk/publications/feeding-minds (accessed 19 January 2022).

Miller, WR and Rollnick, S (1991) *Motivational Interviewing: Preparing People to Change Addictive Behaviour.* New York: Guilford Press.

Miller, WR and Rollnick, S (2002) *Motivational Interviewing: Preparing People for Change* (2nd edition). New York: Guilford Press.

Miller, WR and Rollnick, S (2013) *Motivational Interviewing: Helping People Change* (3rd edition). New York: Guilford Press.

Moos, RH and Schaefer, JA (1984) The crisis of physical illness, in Moos, R (ed.) *Coping with Physical Illness 2: New Perspectives*. New York: Plenum.

Morrison, V and Bennett, P (2006) *An Introduction to Health Psychology*. Harlow: Pearson.

Mortimer, P (2006) Lucy in the sky with diamonds. *Openmind*, July/Aug: 140.

Murphy, R, McGuiness, D, Bainbridge, E et al. (2017) Service users' experiences of involuntary hospital admission under the Mental Health Act 2001 in the Republic of Ireland. *Psychiatric Services*, 68: 1127–35. DOI: 10.1176/appi.ps.201700008

Mustata, AE (2019) Mental health and adverse psychosocial factors in cardiovascular patients. An exploratory and descriptive study. *Journal of Experiential Psychotherapy*, 22 (2): 24–30.

National Institute for Health and Care Excellence (2015) *Violence and Aggression: Short-Term Management in Mental Health, Health and Community Settings. NICE Guideline*. Available online at: www.nice.org.uk/guidance/ng10

National Institute for Mental Health in England (NIMHE) (2005) *NIMHE Guiding Statement on Recovery*. Available online at: https://1library.net/document/z3ov3xez-nimhe-guiding-statement-on-recovery.html

Naylor, C, Das, P, Ross, S, Honeyman, M, Thompson, J and Gilburt, H (2016) *Bringing Together Physical and Mental Health: A New Frontier for Integrated Care*. London: The Kings Fund.

Nazroo, J and Iley, K (2011) Ethnicity, race and mental disorder in the UK, in Pilgrim, D, Rogers, A and Pescosolido, B (eds) *The Sage Handbook of Mental Health and Illness*. London: SAGE.

Nejad, SB, Kargar, A, Hamid, N and Razmjoo, S (2020) Metacognitive beliefs, positive states of mind, and emotional approach coping as the predictors of medical compliance in patients with cancer. *International Journal of Cancer Management*, 13 (7): e101608.

Nelson-Jones, R (2016) *Basic Counselling Skills: A Helper's Guide* (4th edition). London: SAGE.

NHS Business Service Authority (2020) *Medicines Used in Mental Health – England – 2015/16 to 2019/20*. Available online at: www.nhsbsa.nhs.uk/statistical-collections/medicines-used-mental-health-england/medicines-used-mental-health-england-201516-201920

NHS England (2014) *Five Year Forward*. Available online at: www.england.nhs.uk/wp-content/uploads/2014/10/5yfv-web.pdf

Nolan, P and Badger, F (2005) Aspects of the relationship between doctors and depressed patients that enhance satisfaction with primary care. *Journal of Psychiatric and Mental Health Nursing*, 12: 146–53.

Nuffield Council on Bioethics (2009) *Dementia: Ethical Issues*. Available online at: www.nuffieldbioethics.org/wp-content/uploads/2014/07/Dementia-report-Oct-09.pdf

Nursing and Midwifery Council (NMC) (2018a) *Standards Framework for Nursing and Midwifery Education.* Available online at: www.nmc.org.uk/standards-for-education-and-training/standards-framework-for-nursing-and-midwifery-education/

Nursing and Midwifery Council (NMC) (2018b) *Professional Standards of Practice and Behaviour for Nurses, Midwives and Nursing Associates.* Available online at: www.nmc.org.uk/globalassets/sitedocuments/nmc-publications/nmc-code.pdf

Nursing and Midwifery Council (NMC) (2018c) *Future Nurse: Standards of Proficiency for Registered Nurses.* Available online at: www.nmc.org.uk/globalassets/sitedocuments/standards-of-proficiency/nurses/future-nurse-proficiencies.pdf

O'Hagan, M (2014) *Madness Made Me: A Memoir.* Wellington: Open Box.

Park, N, Peterson, C and Seligman, M (2004) Strengths of character and well-being. *Journal of Social and Clinical Psychology,* 23 (5): 603–19.

Paton, F, Wright, K, Ayre, N, Dare, C, Johnson, S, Lloyd-Evans, B et al. (2016) Improving outcomes for people in mental health crisis: A rapid synthesis of the evidence for available models of care. *Health Technology Assessment,* 20 (3). DOI: 10.3310/hta20030

Peplau, H (1952) *Interpersonal Relations in Nursing.* London: Macmillan.

Perkins, R and Morgan, P (2017) Creating recovery-focused services, in Trenoweth, S (ed.) *Promoting Recovery in Mental Health Nursing.* London: Learning Matters.

Perna, R, Rouselle, A and Brennan, P (2003) Traumatic brain injury: Depression, neurogenesis and medication management. *Journal of Head Trauma Rehabilitation,* 18 (2): 201–203.

Peterson, C and Seligman, MEP (2004) *Character Strengths and Virtues: A Handbook and Classification.* New York, NY; Washington, DC: Oxford University Press; American Psychological Association.

Potts, C and Potts, S (2013) *Assertiveness: How to Be Strong in Every Situation.* Chichester: Capstone.

Rassool, G (2000) The crescent and Islam: Healing, nursing and the spiritual dimension. Some considerations towards an understanding of the Islamic perspectives on caring. *Journal of Advanced Nursing,* 32 (6): 1476–84.

Read, JR, Sharpe, L, Modini, M and Dear, BF (2017) Multi-morbidity and depression: A systematic review and meta-analysis. *Journal of Affective Disorders,* 221: 36–46.

Repper, J and Perkins, R (2003) *Social Inclusion and Recovery – A Model for Mental Health Practice.* Edinburgh: Baillière Tindall.

Ridley, J and Hunter, S (2013) Subjective experiences of compulsory treatment from a qualitative study of early implementation of the Mental Health (Care & Treatment) (Scotland) Act 2003. *Health and Social Care in the Community,* 21 (5): 509–18. DOI: 10.1111/hsc.12041

Rogers, A and Pilgrim, D (1994) Service users' views of psychiatric nurses. *British Journal of Nursing,* 3: 16–18.

Rogers, A and Pilgrim, D (2021) *A Sociology of Mental Health and Illness.* London: OUP.

Rogers, C (1951) *Client-Centred Therapy: Its Current Practice, Implications and Theory.* Boston: Houghton Mifflin.

Rotter, JB (1966) Generalized expectancies for internal versus external control of reinforcement. *Psychological Monographs: General and Applied,* 80 (1): 609.

Royal College of Nursing (2020) *First Steps.* Available online at: https://rcni.com/hosted-content/rcn/first-steps/risk-assessment (accessed 28/02/2020).

Royal College of Psychiatrists (2013) *Whole-Person Care: From Rhetoric to Reality. Achieving Parity Between Mental and Physical Health.* Occasional paper. OP88. London: Royal College of Psychiatrists.

Royal Pharmaceutical Society (2016) *A Competency Framework for all Prescribers.* London: Royal Pharmaceutical Society.

Rydon, S (2005) The attitudes, knowledge and skills needed in mental health nurses: The perspective of users of mental health services. *International Journal of Mental Health Nursing,* 14: 78–87.

Ryff, C (1989) Happiness is everything, or is it? Explorations on the meaning of psychological well-being. *Journal of Personality and Social Psychology,* 57: 1069–81.

Ryff, C and Keyes, C (1995) The structure of psychological well-being revisited. *Journal of Personality and Social Psychology,* 69: 719–27.

Sanders, P (2019) Counselling, psychotherapy, diagnosis, and the medicalisation of distress, in Watson, J (ed.) *Drop the Disorder: Challenging the Culture of Psychiatric Diagnosis* (pp. 24–39). Monmouth: PCCS Books.

Sayce, L (2016) *From Psychiatric Patient to Citizen Revisited.* London: Palgrave.

Schreuder, JA, Roelen, CA, Groothoff, JW, van der Klink, JJ, Magerøy, N, Pallesen, S, Bjorvatn, B and Moen, BE (2012) Coping styles relate to health and work environment of Norwegian and Dutch hospital nurses: A comparative study. *Nursing Outlook,* 60 (1): 37–43.

Schwartz, SP, Adair, KC, Bae, J, Rehder, KJ, Shanafelt, TD, Profit, J and Sexton, JB (2019) Work–life balance behaviours cluster in work settings and relate to burnout and safety culture: A cross-sectional survey analysis. *BMJ Quality & Safety,* 28 (2): 142–150.

Seligman, M (2002) *Authentic Happiness.* London: Nicholas Brearley Publishing.

Seligman, M (2008) Positive health. *Applied Psychology: An International Review,* 57: 3–18.

Shattell, M, McAllister, S, Hogan, B and Thomas, S (2006) She took the time to make sure she understood: Mental health patients' experiences of being understood. *Archives of Psychiatric Nursing,* 20 (5): 234–41.

Shedler, J (2010). The efficacy of psychodynamic psychotherapy. *American Psychologist,* 65: 98–109.

Sheerin, F (2019) The cloaked self: Professional decloaking and its implications for human engagement in nursing. *International Journal of Nursing Knowledge,* 30 (2): 99–105. https://doi.org/10.1111/2047-3095.12211

Shepherd, G, Boardman, J and Slade, M (2008) *Making Recovery a Reality.* Available online at: www.centreformentalhealth.org.uk/publications/making-recovery-reality

Skinner, EA and Zimmer-Gembeck, MJ (2016) *The Development of Coping: Stress, Neurophysiology, Social Relationships, and Resilience During Childhood and Adolescence.* Switzerland: Springer.

Slade, M (2009) *Personal Recovery and Mental Illness: A Guide for Mental Health Professionals.* Cambridge: Cambridge University Press.

Snyder, R, Lopez, S and Pedrotti, J (2011) *Positive Psychology: The Scientific and Practical Explorations of Human Strengths* (2nd edition). Thousand Oaks, CA: SAGE.

Stephens, C, Sackett, N, Pierce, R, Schopfer, D, Schmajuk, G, Moy, N, Bachhubber, M, Walhagen, MI and Lee, SJ (2013) Transitional care challenges of rehospitalized veterans: Listening to patients and providers. *Population Health Management*, 16 (5): 326–31.

Stoney, CM, Kaufmann, PG and Czajkowski, SM (2018) Cardiovascular disease: Psychological, social, and behavioral influences: Introduction to the special issue. *American Psychologist*, 73 (8): 949–54.

Sullivan, HS (1953) *The Interpersonal Theory of Psychiatry.* London: WW Norton.

Swinton, J (2001) *Spirituality and Mental Health Care.* London: Jessica Kingsley.

Taylor, DM, Barnes, T and Young, A (2021) *The Maudsley Prescribing Guidelines in Psychiatry* (14th edition). Chichester: Wiley Blackwell.

Taylor, TL, Hawton, K, Fortune, S and Kapur, N (2009) Attitudes towards clinical services among people who self-harm: Systematic review. *British Journal of Psychiatry*, 194: 104–10.

The Mental Health Taskforce (2016) *The Five Year Forward View for Mental Health.* Available online at: www.england.nhs.uk/wp-content/uploads/2016/02/Mental-Health-Taskforce-FYFV-final.pdf

Todres, L, Galvin, K and Holloway, I (2009) The humanisation of health: A value framework for qualitative research. *International Journal of Qualitative Studies on Health and Wellbeing*, 1–10.

Trenoweth, S (2003) Perceiving risk in dangerous situations. *Journal of Advanced Nursing*, 42 (3): 278–87.

Trenoweth, S, Tingle, A and Clark, T (2017) What is recovery? in Trenoweth, S (ed.) *Promoting Recovery in Mental Health Nursing.* London: Learning Matters.

Tronto, JC (2013) *Caring Democracy, Markets, Equality and Justice.* New York: University Press.

Tyson, PJ (2013) A service user-initiated project investigating the attitudes of mental health staff towards clients and services in an acute mental health unit. *Journal of Psychiatric and Mental Health Nursing*, 20: 379–386.

Üzar-Özçetin, S, Tee, S and Trenoweth, S (2021) Achieving culturally competent mental health care: A mixed-method study drawing on the perspectives of UK nursing students. *Perspectives in Psychiatric Care*, DOI: 10.1111/ppc.12926.

Van der Kolk, B (2014) *The Body Keeps the Score: Mind, Brain, and Body in Transformation of Trauma.* London: Penguin.

van der Wardt, V, di Lorito, C and Viniol, A (2021) Promoting physical activity in primary care: A systematic review and meta-analysis. *British Journal of General Practice*, 71 (706): e399–405. https://doi.org/10.3399/BJGP.2020.0817

Ventegodt, S and Merrick, J (2013) *Textbook on Evidence-Based Holistic Mind–Body Medicine: Basic Philosophy and Ethics of Traditional Hippocratic Medicine*. New York: Nova Science Publishers.

Vollenweider, P, Waeber, G, Bastardot, F and Preisig, M (2011) Cardiovascular disease and mental disorders: Bidirectional risk factors. *Cardiovascular Diseases and Mental Disorders*, 1 (3): 63–6.

Waddill-Goad, S and Sigma Theta Tau International (2016) *Nurse Burnout: Overcoming Stress in Nursing*. Indianapolis, IN: Sigma Theta Tau International.

Walker, MT (2006) The social construction of mental illness and its implications for the recovery model. *The International Journal of Psychosocial Rehabilitation*, 10 (1): 71–87.

Walker, S (2017) How do patients who have self-harmed experience contact with mental health services in a general hospital?: An exploratory study using Interpretative Phenomenological Analysis. Unpublished thesis, University of Southampton.

Walker, S, Kennedy, A, Vassilev, I and Rogers, A (2017) How do people with long-term mental health problems negotiate relationships with network members at times of crisis? *Health Expectations*, 1–11.

Wallston, KA, Wallston, BS and DeVellis, R (1978) Development of the multidimensional health locus of control (MHLOC) scale. *Health Education Monographs*, 6: 161–70.

Warner, R (1985) *Recovery from Schizophrenia: Psychiatry and Political Economy*. London: Routledge and Kegan Paul.

Watkins, P (2001) *Mental Health Nursing: The Art of Compassionate Care*. Edinburgh: Butterworth Heinemann.

Watson, JB and Rayner, R (1920) Conditioned emotional reactions. *Journal of Experimental Psychology*, 3 (1): 1–14.

Waugh, A and Grant, A (2018) *Ross and Wilson Anatomy and Physiology in Health and Illness* (13th ed.). Edinburgh: Elsevier.

Weary, G and Edwards, JA (1996) Causal uncertainty and related goal structures, in Sorrentino, R and Higgins, ET (eds) *The Handbook of Motivation and Cognition* (Vol. 3): *The Interpersonal Context* (pp. 148–81). New York: Guilford.

Weary, G, Jacobson, JA, Edwards, JA and Tobin, SJ (2001) Chronic and temporarily activated causal uncertainty beliefs and stereotype usage. *Journal of Personality and Social Psychology*, 81: 206–19.

Woods, SB, Priest, JB and Denton, WH (2015) Tell me where it hurts: Assessing mental and relational health in primary care using a biopsychosocial assessment intervention. *Family Journal*, 23 (2). DOI: 10.1177/1066480714555671

World Health Organization (WHO) (1946) *Constitution of the World Health Organization*. Available online at: www.who.int/governance/eb/who_constitution_en.pdf (accessed 19 January 2022).

References

World Health Organization (WHO) (2001) *AUDIT: The Alcohol Use Disorders Identification Test: Guidelines for Use in Primary Health Care* (2nd edition). Available online at: https://apps.who.int/iris/handle/10665/67205

World Health Organization (WHO) (2018) *Mental Health: Strengthening Our Response.* Available online at: www.who.int/news-room/fact-sheets/detail/mental-health-strengthening-our-response

World Health Organization (2019) *International Classification of Diseases for Mortality and Morbidity Statistics* (11th revision). Available online at: https://icd.who.int/browse11/l-m/en

Yerkes, R and Dodson, J (1908) The relation of strength of stimulus to rapidity of habit-formation. *Journal of Comparative Neurology and Psychology*, 18 (5): 459–82.

Zubin, J and Spring, B (1977) Vulnerability: A new view of schizophrenia. *Journal of Abnormal Psychology*, 86 (2): 103–26.

Zuckerman, M (2009) Sensation seeking. In Leary, MR and Hoyle, RH (eds.). *Handbook of Individual Differences in Social Behavior* (pp. 455–65). New York: Guilford Press.

Index

Locators in **bold** refer to tables and those in *italics* to figures.